The Ageless B8dy

How to Remain a Human Dynamo and Retain a Perfect Physique —With The Magic of Kettlebells

ANDREA DU CANE

MASTER RKC INSTRUCTOR

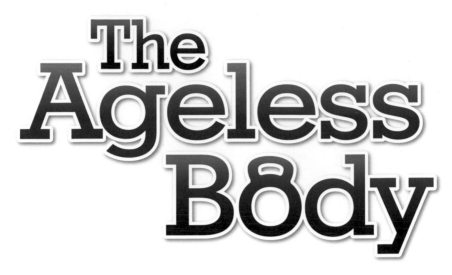

The Ageless B8dy

How to Remain a Human Dynamo and Retain a Perfect Physique —With The Magic of Kettlebells

ANDREA DU CANE
MASTER RKC INSTRUCTOR

Published in the United States by:
Dragon Door Publications, Inc
P.O. Box 4381, St. Paul, MN 55104
Tel: (651) 487-2180 • Fax: (651) 487-3954
Credit card orders: 1-800-899-5111
Email: dragondoor@aol.com • Website: www.dragondoor.com

ISBN 10: 0-938045-81-4   ISBN 13: 978-0-938045-81-6

This edition first published in January, 2012

Printed in China

Book design, and cover by Derek Brigham, Site: www.dbrigham.com • (763) 208-3069 • Email: bigd@dbrigham.com
Photography: Don Pitlik (main photography) and Chas Jensen (gym stretching images)

To John and Pat Du Cane,

For entering your 90th year with humor, joy, and strength.
You have been an inspiration to me
for the strength you bring to perseverance,
for the courage in which you face adversity,
and for the boundless joy you bring to embracing life.

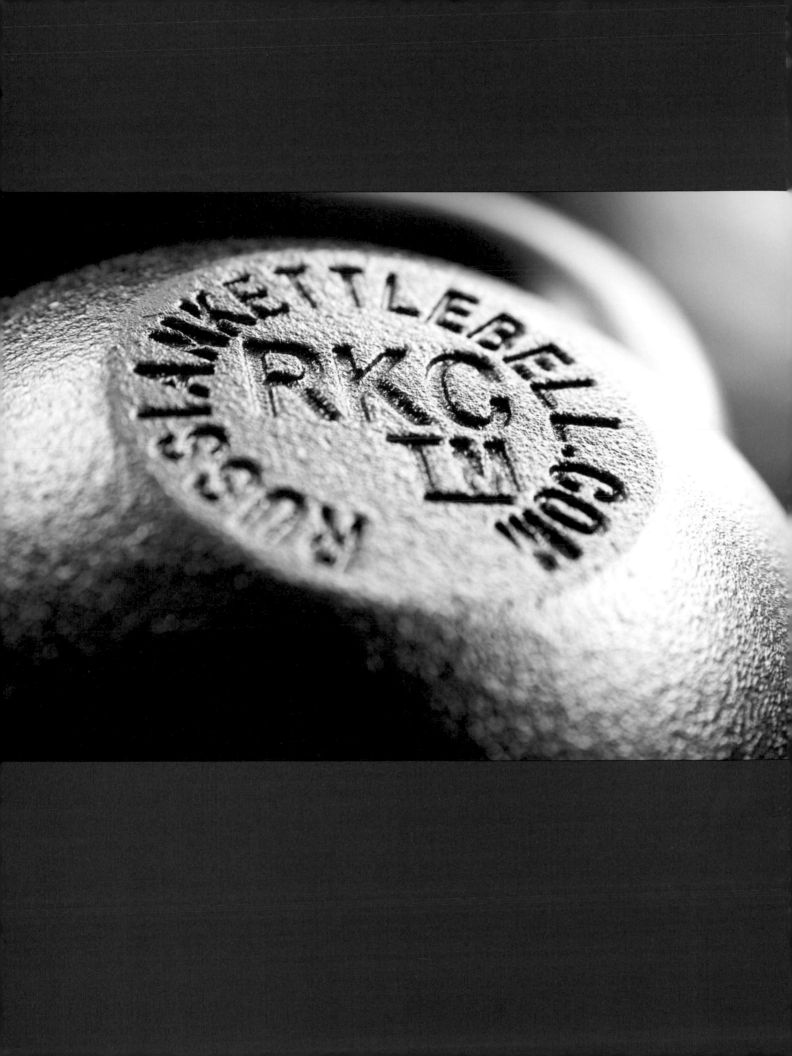

TABLE OF CONTENTS

Preface V

Part I: Before You Begin
Chapter 1
Introduction...1
Common Questions 1
How to Use This Book 3

Chapter 2
Medical Disclaimer 5

Chapter 3
Kettlebell Safety 7
Types of Injuries 7
Support Structures 7

Chapter 4
Self Screen 9
Shoulder Mobility Screen........................9
Hip Mobility Screen..............................12

Part II: Drills and Exercises
Chapter 5
Prep Drills..19
Neutral Spine..19
Hip Hinge 22
Hip Flexor Stretch.................................26
T-Spine Rotation 28
Seated Push/Pull...................................30

Chapter 6
Warm-Up Exercises 33
Three-Way Neck Movements 33
Arm and Shoulder Movements 37
Torso and Pelvis Movements 41
Elbow, Wrist, and Finger Movements 44
Leg and Foot Movements 49

Chapter 7
Main Kettlebell Exercises........................53
Deadlift..53
Carry 62
Plank...65
Swing..68
Press...72
Goblet Squat 77
Russian Twist 81

Chapter 8
The Get-Up 85

Chapter 9
Balance Drills.................................93
No Weight, Using a Chair 93
Holding the Kettlebell at the Side..............95
Holding the Kettlebell
    in the Clean Position.......................95
Holding the Kettlebell Overhead................96

Chapter 10
Cool-Down Stretches 97
Hip Flexor Stretch.............................97
Half-Pigeon/Figure 4 100
Quad Stretch...................................103
Hamstring Stretch 105
T-Spine Rotation 108
Seated Push/Pull...............................110
Down Dog.......................................112

Chapter 11
Advanced Kettlebell Exercises..............115
Clean..115
Double Swing 118
Double Clean 120
Double Press 122
Front Squat....................................124
Goblet Squat with a Curl 125
Goblet Squat with a Front Raise 126
Snatch 127

Part III: Workouts

Chapter 12
Planning Your Workouts.....................131

Chapter 13
**Six-Week Ramp-Up &
Six-Week Program** 133
Preparatory and Instructional Phase 134
Sample Six-Week Program:
Overall Strength And Conditioning 136

Chapter 14
Strength Workout 139
Round 1..139
Round 2..140
Round 3..140
Round 4..141
Round 5..141
Round 6..142

Chapter 15
Cardio Workout 143
Round 1..143
Round 2..144
Round 3..144
Round 4..145
Round 5..145
Round 6..146
Round 7..146
Round 8..146

Resources 147
References 148
About the Author 149

Preface

The inspiration for *The Ageless Body* book and DVD began back in early 2002. Now, almost 10 years later, I can't believe it has taken me so long to reach a group of people who not only deserve such a training program, attention, and empowerment but who also need these things so much.

The story really began on the day I picked up my first kettlebell. We had been photographing Pavel doing a few "ab" exercises for an upcoming book when I saw the kettlebells hiding over in the corner. The only thing I could do with them was a deadlift. I thought they were very interesting, but it was hard for me to envision doing much with them.

Later, as more books came out—including, finally, Pavel's *Russian Kettlebell Challenge*—I began to ask, "Why aren't there kettlebells for women to use?" (At that time, kettlebells came in only the 16 kg, 24 kg, and 32 kg sizes.) It didn't take too long before Pavel agreed to do a book and DVD for women, which became *From Russia with Tough Love*.

About a week before filming, I received my first kettlebell. It was 18 lbs. I can't tell you how excited I was! This was MY kettlebell. It was made for me—a woman. I could press it and snatch it and do swings and windmills. It was AWESOME!

I distinctly remember thinking, "This is what every woman should do." Every person—not just tough military guys, law enforcement officers, and martial artists—but all people should have access to this incredible tool. My background in dance, martial arts, and Pilates allowed me to see the kettlebell's overall health benefits and how this simple hunk of iron could turn into an incredible tool of healing for all people.

I decided to bring the kettlebell experience to a broader female market, and so *The Kettlebell Goddess Workout* DVD materialized. I intended to make that DVD as interactive as possible, while still keeping the program design simple. It has achieved all that I hoped it would. That DVD has reached out to many women who may not have had the courage or desire to pick up a kettlebell before.

I truly believe that kettlebell training is for everyone. It can be for people coming back from injury, for those who are deconditioned, and, of course, for the elderly. I have spent the last couple years of my career focusing on the needs of people with specific limitations and special issues. For example, my DVD *Working with Special Populations* was filmed at an RKC Level II certification and was designed specifically to help trainers who are teaching kettlebells to clients with limitations.

Since release of the *Special Populations* and *Goddess* DVDs, I have received questions from many people asking me how they can get their mothers, fathers, grandparents, and sedentary friends started with kettlebells. I'm aware that this group has been underserved in the kettlebell world. Until now, no product has been aimed at them. Working with them may not be as glamorous as working with competitive athletes and military personnel, but I feel so much satisfaction from knowing that I have helped change a life. If I can make just one person feel stronger, move better, or have less pain in his or her day-to-day life, then I have achieved my goal.

I want to emphasize that *The Ageless Body* book and DVD are not just for seniors and aging athletes. Young people and those inexperienced with kettlebells will also benefit from the safe, simple, and progressive format that this program provides. The screens and modifications provided by the program will allow people of any skill level to begin their kettlebell program and to advance at their own pace.

My own journey with kettlebells continues, even as a Master RKC Instructor. I hope that this book and DVD will be the start of your own wonderful journey. May that journey be filled with accomplishment, improved health and strength, and continued enjoyment of life.

SPECIAL THANKS

I would like to thank the hard-working staff at Dragon Door—Nicole Du Cane and Timothy Spencer—for lending their time and talents to the development and production of this book.

And most importantly, I would like to thank Pavel Tsatsouline for "Pavelizing" the fitness industry and for personally encouraging me to reach out with our "Hard Style School of Strength" to empower the boomer and senior populations.

Andrea Du Cane

Andrea Du Cane

Master RKC Instructor

Part I
Before You Begin

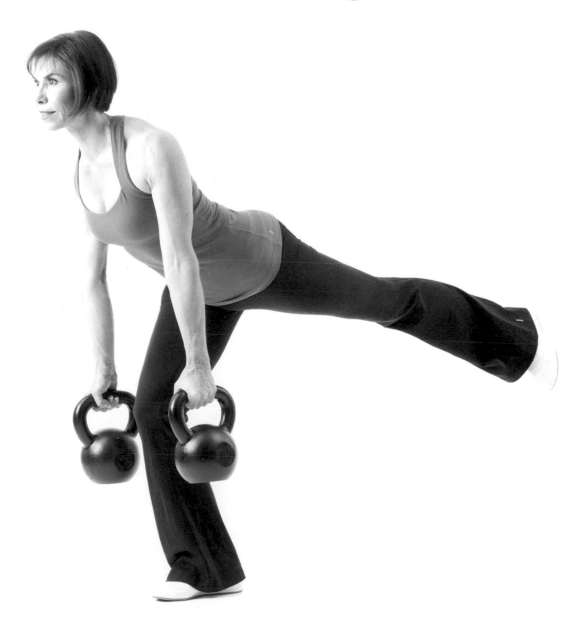

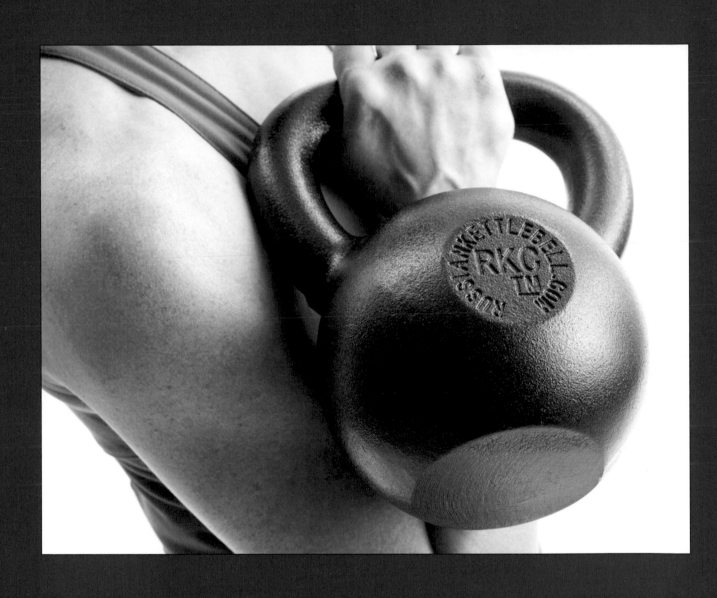

Chapter 1

Introduction

The Ageless Body program is designed to take you to a new level of health and fitness. It's organized so that no matter where you are starting from, you will achieve a level of fitness that will allow you to continue to pursue your favorite activities and enjoy your daily life.

This book has everything you need to start training with kettlebells. It's instructional but also contains two workouts: one focusing on strength and the other on conditioning.

Make sure you read this introductory section thoroughly. It contains what you need to know to get started, including discussions of footwear and platforms, what size kettlebell to use, and which level to follow.

COMMON QUESTIONS

Why is strength training important?

To begin, it's important to make the distinction between physiological age and chronological age. We can't do anything about our chronological age, but we do have the power to make certain lifestyle choices that can help keep us young. Strength training is a huge part of this. It can turn back the hands of time and help us look and feel younger as we get into our 50s, 60s, 70s, and beyond.

One of the biggest problems with getting older is the loss of muscle and strength, which is called sarcopenia. In physically inactive people, about 0.5% of lean muscle mass is lost every year between the ages of 25 and 60. From age 60 on, the rate of loss doubles to about 1% per year. It doubles again at age 70, again at age 80, and then again at age 90.

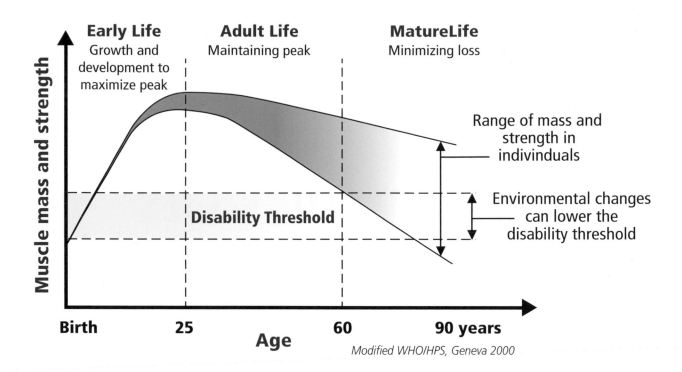

Early Life
Growth and development to maximize peak

Adult Life
Maintaining peak

MatureLife
Minimizing loss

Muscle mass and strength

Range of mass and strength in individuals

Environmental changes can lower the disability threshold

Disability Threshold

Birth   25   60   90 years

Age

Modified WHO/HPS, Geneva 2000

Sarcopenia can be thought of as the muscular equivalent to *osteoporosis*—the loss of bone—which is also caused by inactivity. The combination of osteoporosis and sarcopenia results in the significant frailty often seen in elderly individuals.

In advanced age, the lack of muscular strength becomes the inability to get up from a chair without bracing yourself with your arms, the loss of mobility means no more squatting down or bending over to put pans away on the lowest shelves, and the deterioration of balance makes just stepping out of the bathtub a risk. For nonseniors, these factors can show up in a weakened golf swing, trouble picking up the grandkids, and even difficulty balancing on one foot.

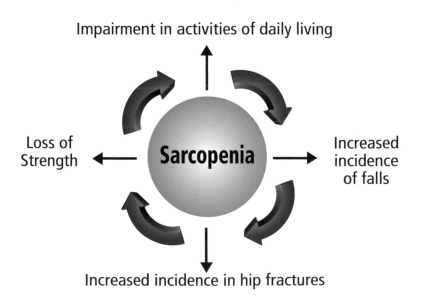

Impairment in activities of daily living

Loss of Strength

Sarcopenia

Increased incidence of falls

Increased incidence in hip fractures

Let's face it: You need strength, mobility, and balance (in every sense of the word) to lead an active, healthy, and productive life.

Fortunately, sarcopenia can be stopped and even reversed with strength training. Strength training leads to an increase in lean body mass and to a decrease in fat. For every 10 pounds of lean body mass we carry, 500 calories is expended per day to maintain that mass. Being lean is like having your own fat-burning "furnace."

Eating well, getting regular exercise, taking the right supplements, and learning how to deal with stress are all ways to stay young. All of them will have a positive impact on everything from your blood pressure and resting heart rate to your body weight, muscle mass, and triglyceride levels. Taking these steps will also go a long way in controlling diseases such as diabetes, heart disease, and even cancer.

I'm not saying that following a healthy lifestyle will cure any of these diseases, but it will help prevent some of the typical signs of aging.

Why kettlebells and not other types of strength training?

It's all in the design. The kettlebell is the only hand-held weight that can be used aerobically for cardio, as well as anaerobically for strength training. The handle allows for the weight to be offset, adding a unique resistance to every movement you do and allowing your muscles to work through a greater range of motion. It's the only training tool that allows you to get a complete, full body, strength and conditioning workout all at the same time. We like to call the kettlebell a "gym in your hand."

HOW TO USE THIS BOOK

Before beginning either workout in this book, read through the entire Part I. In particular, you must complete the Self-Screen to determine which level is appropriate for you (see Chapter 4). Once you have completed the Self-Screen, you will be ready to move on to Part II, the instructional section.

In that section, you will begin with the Prep Drills (see Chapter 5). They are designed to help you learn about your body's alignment and position and to prepare your shoulders for the mobility that's required for the overhead lifts. Being able to perform these basic drills is essential for performing the more complex exercises later on. Please complete and familiarize yourself with all the Prep Drills before moving on to the Main Kettlebell Exercises (see Chapter 7).

Chapter 7, Main Kettlebell Exercises, contains all the exercises found in the workouts. It's vital that you learn the proper form for all of the exercises *first*, so you can perform them safely during the workout. You may spend the first week or two working on just one drill. Remember that you need *to practice them to master them!* You MUST feel confident in all the drills before you do the actual workout.

Part II also contains two special sections: one focusing on the get-up (Chapter 8) and the other on balance (Chapter 9). The get-up is a foundational exercise in the kettlebell training system known as the RKC (Russian Kettlebell Challenge). Performing this exercise teaches you how to stabilize your shoulder while moving from the floor to a standing position, along with how to safely get up from and down to the ground.

Chapter 9, Balance Drills, will help you develop the strength to stand on one leg while holding a kettlebell in different positions. Balance is a big problem not only for seniors but also, remarkably, for people of all ages and backgrounds—even those who may appear to be very fit. Nobody has an excuse! Balance and stability must be trained.

I have also included a warm-up and a cool-down to be followed with every workout. The warm-up exercises in Chapter 6 are designed to warm up the muscles, joints, and nervous system, preparing you for the workout. Even if you plan on just doing one exercise, warming up is essential. After working out it is important that you allow your body to cool down and slowly recover. The stretching exercises are meant to minimize muscle soreness and improve flexibility.

Part III provides two main workouts—one with a strength focus (Chapter 14) and the other with cardio (Chapter 15)—and there are four different levels for each exercise. Pick the level that's right for you for each particular exercise, and don't forget that you can switch levels throughout the workout.

The workout sections are broken down into rounds, and each round is timed. If you are using the book without the DVD, make sure you have a stopwatch, timer, or Gymboss handy to time your sets. Using timed sets allows you to perform the exercises at your own pace.

Some rounds will have multiple exercises, and some will have only one. Some exercises will be repeated during a round. Most rounds will be timed at 30-second intervals. Where the text specifies a 1:1 work-to-rest ratio, that means that you will work for 30 seconds, rest for 30 seconds, and then repeat. If you are training with a partner, one of you should work while the other rests.

Some rounds specify "No rest," which means that you must go through one exercise for the prescribed time and then immediately transition to the next exercise. Going through both exercises one time each in a "No rest" format constitutes the completion of one set.

Stop at *any time* if you need to rest or take a break. If you are not feeling confident about a certain section, just skip it and move on the next round.

Chapter 2

Medical Disclaimer

To do the Ageless Body program, you must be completely cleared by your doctor, especially your cardiologist and orthopedist, and you must have completed any necessary physical therapy. Kettlebell training can be intense, so you need to monitor your heart rate.

Those of you with hip and knee replacements need to check with your doctor on any limitations you may have. Generally, with a hip replacement, there is a 90° limit on hip flexion. You will notice in some of the photos that I'm using a small block to raise the kettlebell, allowing me to keep within a 90° angle. Completing the Self-Screen will help you determine if you need to use a platform, whether or not you have a hip or knee replacement. For some exercises, you will want to follow the "Beginner" version; for example, instead of the goblet squat, you will do the box squat.

Certain breathing techniques, including power breathing, may not be appropriate for people with heart problems or high blood pressure. Please check with your doctor.

I highly recommend seeking out a certified RKC instructor or a CK-FMS (Certified Kettlebell–Functional Movement Specialist) prior to or along with using this book and DVD. You can only learn so much from a book and DVD, and having a trained expert watch your form is invaluable for safe and effective training. At the Resources section at the end of this book, I provide information to help you find instructors in your area.

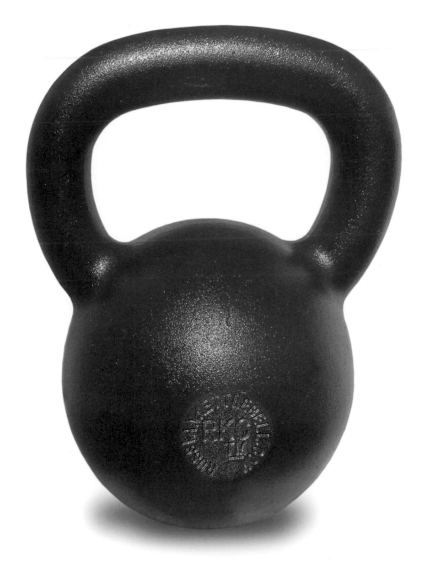

Chapter 3

Kettlebell Safety

- Always be aware of your surroundings!

- Train on a flat surface, where you won't be afraid to drop the kettlebell if something goes wrong.

- Keep pets and small children out of the way.

- Wear proper shoes, or go barefoot. You will notice that I'm wearing flat-soled martial arts shoes. Other good options are Converse Chuck Taylors, Pumas, and Vibram FiveFingers.

- Practice good form with every rep. It's quality, not quantity, that matters. Also, don't forget to monitor your fatigue, and stop when you lose form or concentration.

- Make sure you are breathing! Don't hold your breath. If you can't catch your breath or your heart starts racing, carefully put down the kettlebell and walk around until your breath and heart rate come back down to normal.

- Don't just stop when you finish your sets. Keep moving while your heart rate is still high.

- Watch your posture at the end of your training. Don't slouch or bend forward to catch your breath. It's much safer for your lower back to do gentle back bends or stand up tall while your body is cooling down.

- Build up in repetitions and weight very slowly! You need to allow time for your body's connective tissue to catch up with gains in muscle strength and to allow your mobility a chance to increase, allowing for safe muscle loading.

• Certain breathing techniques, including power breathing, may not be appropriate for people with heart problems or high blood pressure. Please check with your doctor.

• Stop immediately if you feel any abnormal or unusual pain; such as sharp, shooting pain in your lower back, down your leg or in your chest.

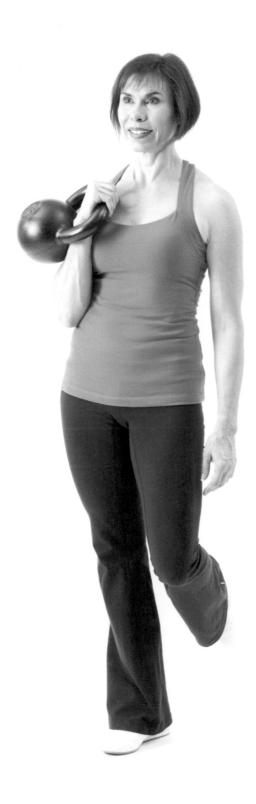

Chapter 4

Self Screen

SHOULDER MOBILITY SCREEN

Key Points:

1. Standing, lock your elbow at your side.

2. Maintaining a straight arm, slowly raise your arm overhead.

3. Your elbow must remain locked and your shoulder down.

4. If your arm does not reach your nose, you will follow level 1.

5. If your arm reaches between your nose and ear, you will follow level 2.

6. If one or both arms reach your ear, you will follow level 3 or 4.

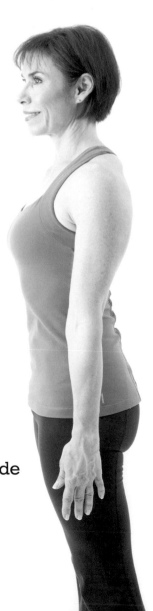

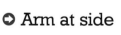 Arm at side

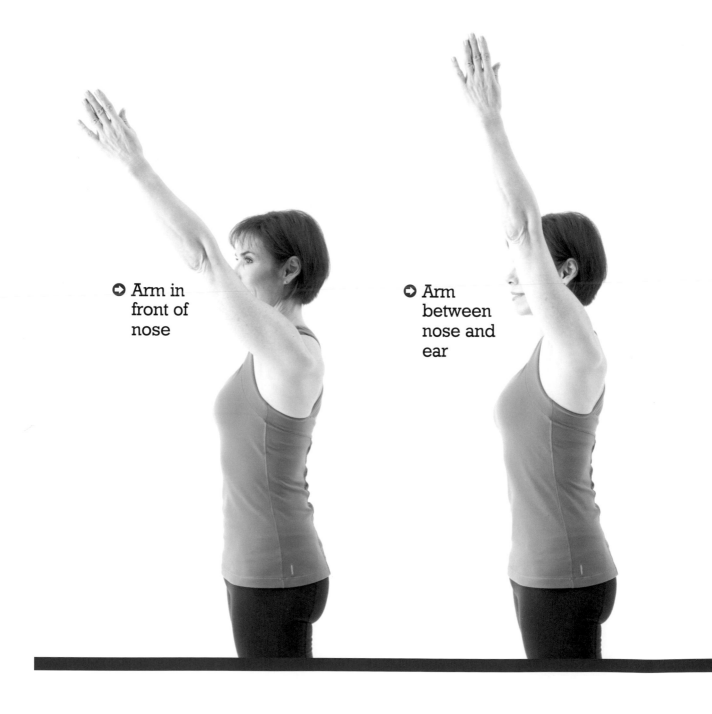

➲ Arm in
front of
nose

➲ Arm
between
nose and
ear

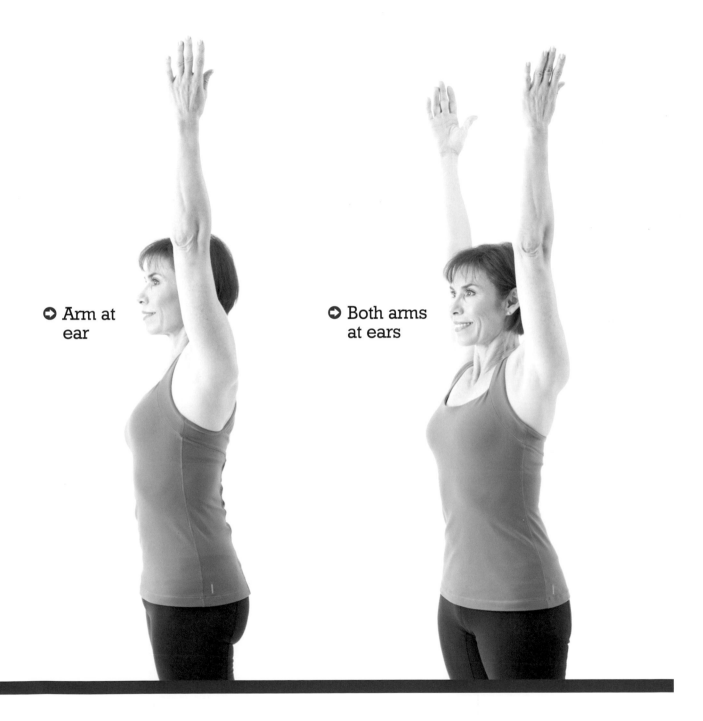

● Arm at ear

● Both arms at ears

HIP MOBILITY SCREEN
Key Points:

1. Stand with your feet hip distance apart, toes straight ahead.

2. Keeping your knees straight, slowly bend forward and reach for your toes.

3. If you can touch your toes or the floor, you will not need to use a platform.

4. If you cannot touch your toes, you will need to use a platform.

● Touching floor

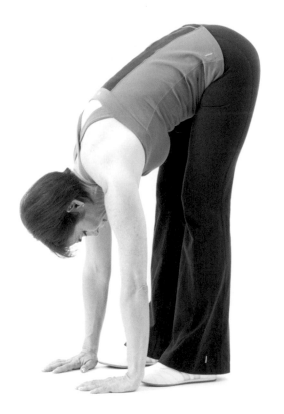

● Hands at ankles

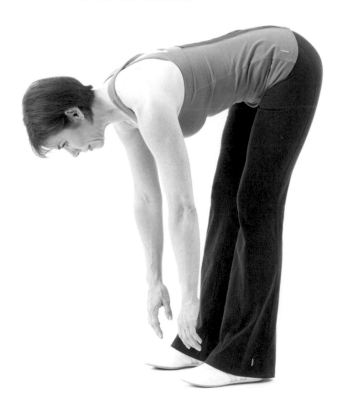

● Hands at knees

● Hands at shins

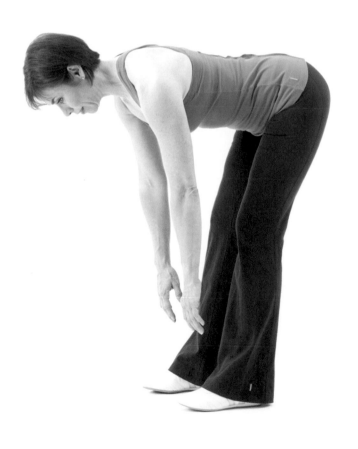

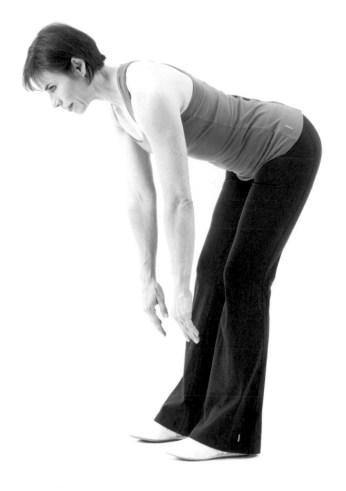

Note: If you can't touch your toes, you will need to raise your kettlebell off the floor using a platform. The height of the platform will depend on the depth of your toe touch. Match the height of the platform to the distance from your fingertips to the floor. A good rule of thumb is to have the handle of the kettlebell at the same height as where your hands reached during the hip mobility screen.

You will need to find a platform or box that matches your level of flexibility. Here are some examples of items you can use from around the house:

- Small stool
- Yoga block
- Hardcover dictionary
- Sturdy block of wood
- Aerobic step

○ Suitcase DL position

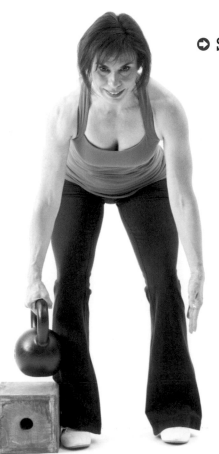
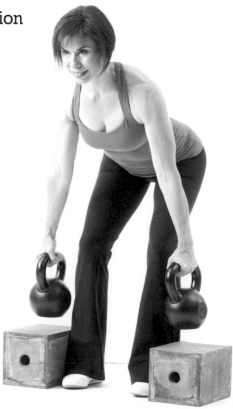

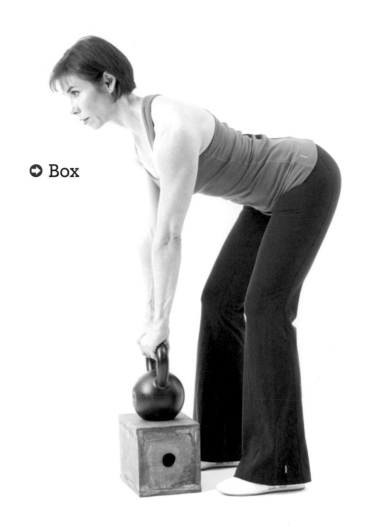

➲ Box

➲ Hard cover dictionary

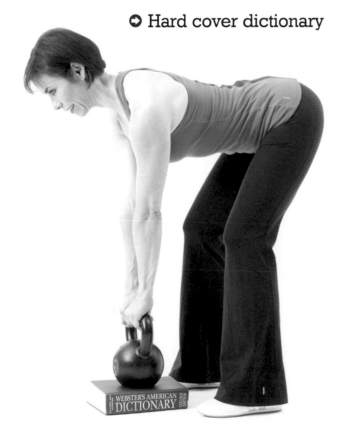

➲ From floor

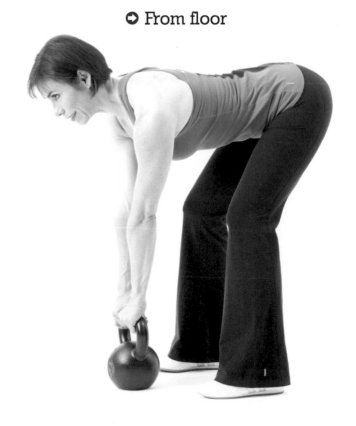

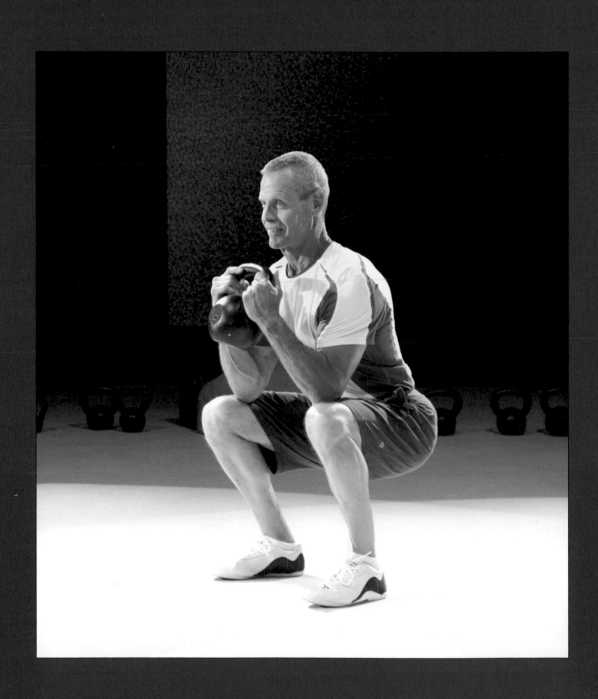

Part II
Drills and
Exercises

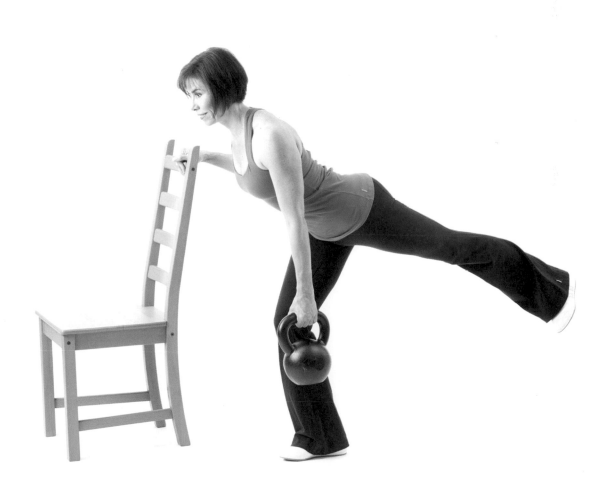

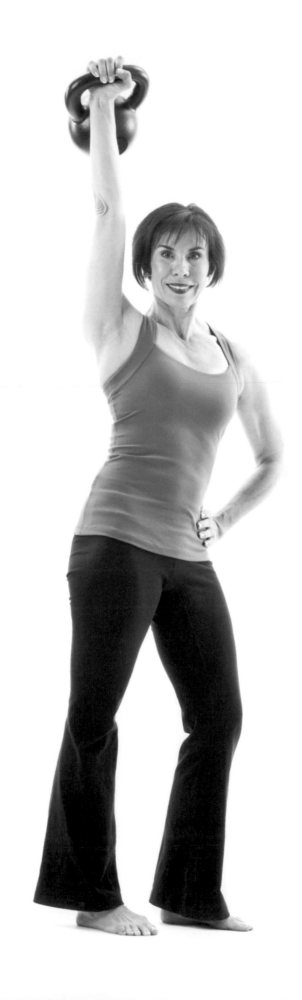

Chapter 5

Prep Drills

NEUTRAL SPINE

Key Points:

1. Stand with your feet hip distance apart, with your side facing a mirror, if possible. Place one hand on the front of your hip bone and the other back. (Placing your hand on your hip, slide your thumb toward your spine and feel for a bony knob. That's what you are looking for.)

2. While watching yourself in the mirror, adjust your front fingers and your back fingers to be level. You have just found your *neutral pelvis.*

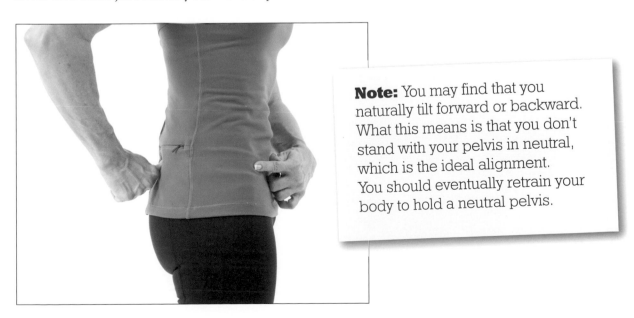

Note: You may find that you naturally tilt forward or backward. What this means is that you don't stand with your pelvis in neutral, which is the ideal alignment. You should eventually retrain your body to hold a neutral pelvis.

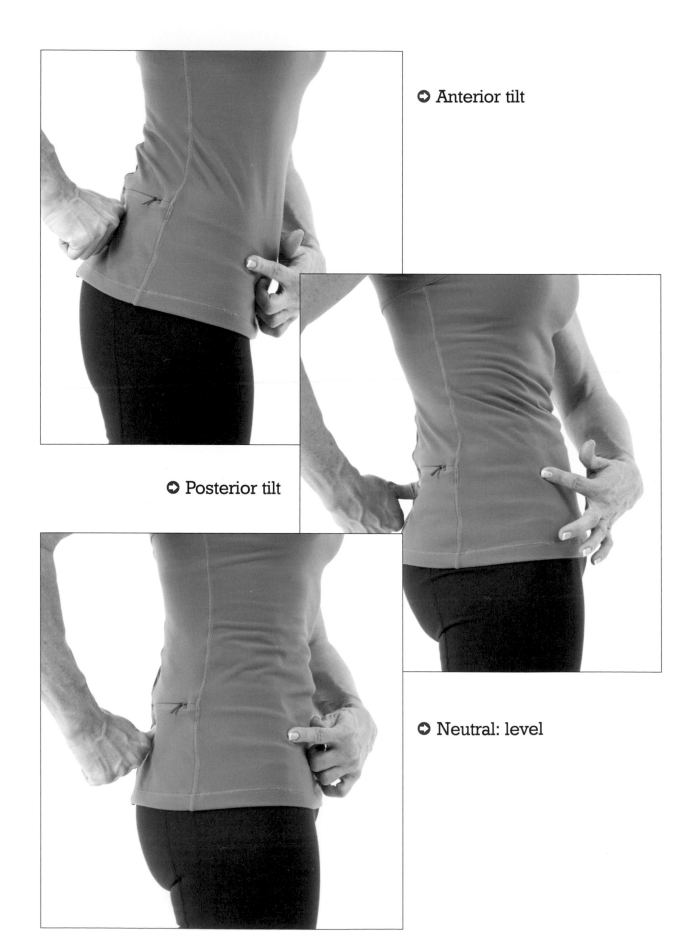

○ Anterior tilt

○ Posterior tilt

○ Neutral: level

Neutral Spine from Deadlift or Hip-Hinge Position

Key Points:

1. From standing, with your pelvis in neutral, notice the natural curve in your lower back. Place your hand there, and feel the curve.

2. Bend forward, keeping the curve. Feel how you have to push your hips backward to maintain the curve.

3. Now place your hands on top of your thighs for support, and rock your pelvis forward. Your lower back should rise up and round out. Notice how your glutes get softer; they should feel less pull or tension. You might also notice more tightness in your lower back.

4. Rock your pelvis in the opposite direction. You should regain your lower-back curve and feel your hamstrings and glutes get tighter. The tightness in your lower back should have gone away.

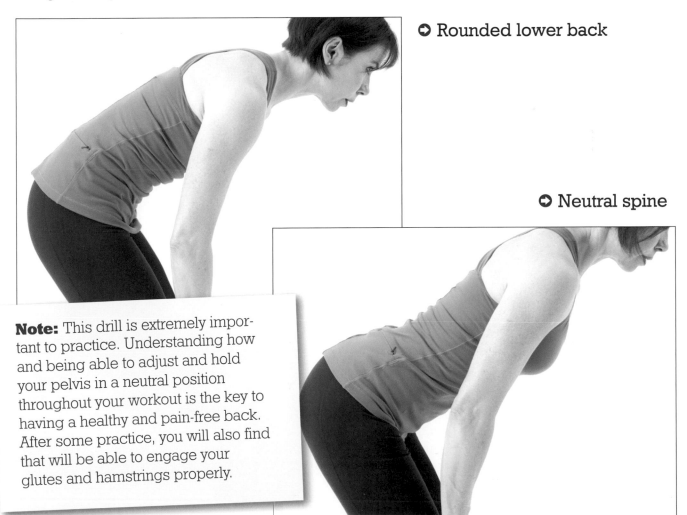

➡ Rounded lower back

➡ Neutral spine

Note: This drill is extremely important to practice. Understanding how and being able to adjust and hold your pelvis in a neutral position throughout your workout is the key to having a healthy and pain-free back. After some practice, you will also find that will be able to engage your glutes and hamstrings properly.

HIP HINGE
Using Hands
Key Points:

1. Stand with your feet hip distance apart, feet straight ahead.

2. Push your hips straight back, placing the edges of your hands in the creases at the tops of your thighs.

3. Use your hands to push your hips back.

4. Keep your spine in neutral, or slightly arch your back.

5. Hinge at the hips, your torso moving forward and your hips moving back.

6. Your spine should stay straight, but your torso will lean forward to face the ground.

7. Bring your hips back forward to return to the starting position.

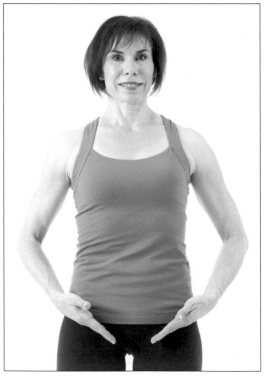

➲ Standing with hands in crease

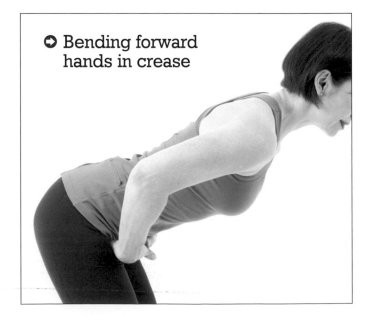

➲ Bending forward hands in crease

Using a Stick
Key Points:

1. Hold a dowel or a broomstick against your back.

2. Use one hand to hold the stick behind your neck, your palm facing your neck. Place your other hand at your lower back, your palm facing behind you.

3. Make sure the stick is touching at the back of your head, between your shoulder blades, and near your tailbone.

4. Bend forward, as in the first hip hinge.

5. The stick must keep contact with the three points on your body throughout the movement.

6. Keep your knees soft to allow your hips to move backward.

7. Bring your hips forward to return to the starting position.

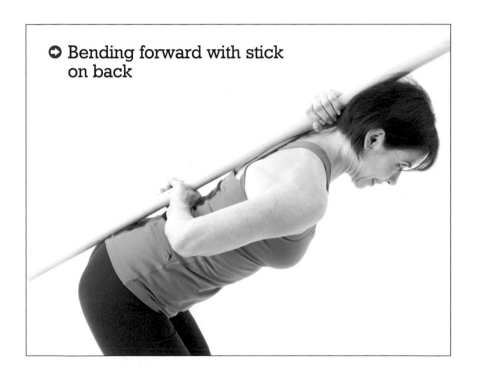

➲ Bending forward with stick on back

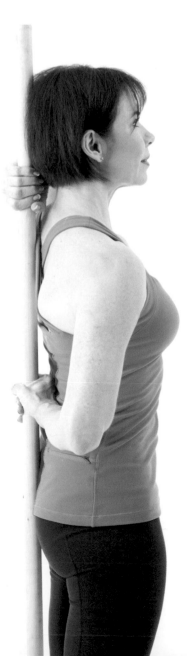

➲ Standing with stick on back

Using a Chair
Key Points:

1. Grab on to a high-backed, sturdy chair with both hands.

2. Place your feet hip distance apart.

3. Push your hips back.

4. Keep your arms straight

5. Let your knees bend as much as needed.

6. Keep your head in line with your back.

7. Bring your hips forward to return to the starting position.

⊙ Bending forward
hands on chair

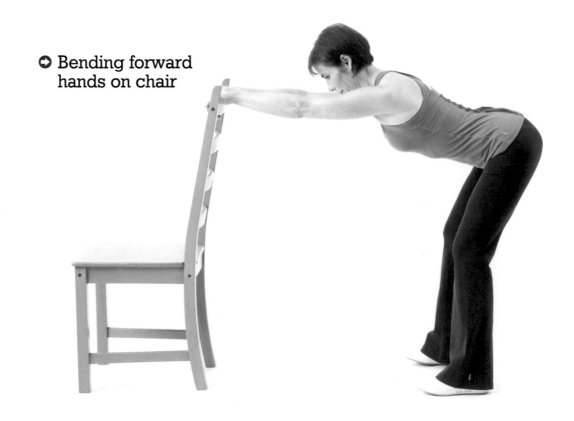

Using a Wall and Chair
Key Points:

1. Stand with your back to a wall that's about 1 foot away.

2. Have a high-backed chair in front of and facing away from you.

3. Hang on to the back of the chair, with your arms straight.

4. Push your hips back to touch the wall.

5. Keep your spine neutral and lengthened.

6. Move your hands down the chair to go deeper, but maintain your back alignment.

7. Bring your hips forward to return to the starting position.

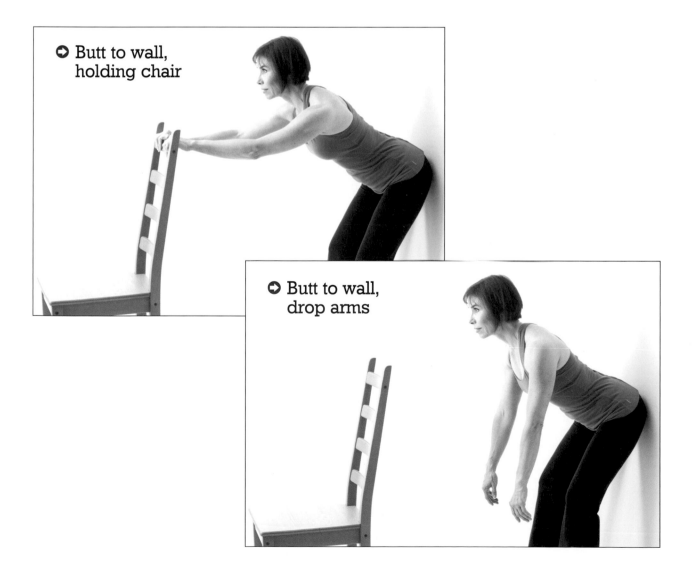

➲ Butt to wall, holding chair

➲ Butt to wall, drop arms

HIP FLEXOR STRETCH
Key Points:

1. Start by kneeling with one leg forward on a soft surface, your hips squared straight ahead and level.

2. Your legs should be hip distance apart and follow imaginary parallel lines.

3. Place your hands on your hips or the small of your back.

4. Squeeze your glutes and push forward with your pelvis, simultaneously reaching your head to the ceiling and lengthening your spine.

5. Do not allow your forward knee to travel over your toes.

6. Keep your eyes level, or look slightly up.

7. Exhale as you go forward, and inhale as you come back up. Repeat a few times, moving in and out of the stretch in a gentle rhythm.

8. Repeat using your other leg.

⊃ Standing using a chair

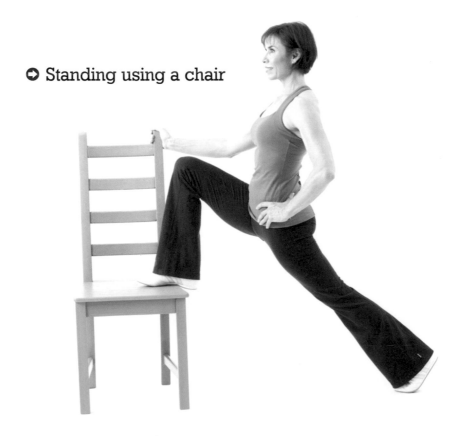

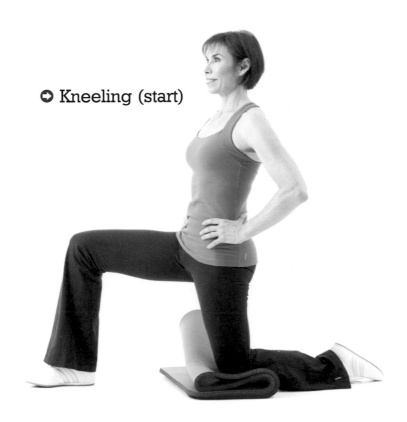

➲ Kneeling (start)

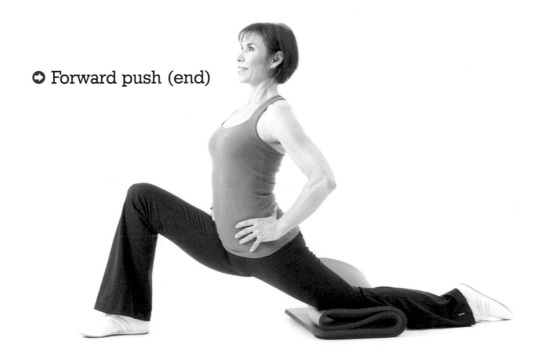

➲ Forward push (end)

T-SPINE ROTATION
Key Points:

1. Lay on the floor on your right side. Bring both knees toward your chest, and then hold them to the ground with your right hand.

2. With your left hand, reach across your chest to grab hold of your ribcage.

3. Turn your head and look left with your eyes, pulling your chest left and open as you exhale.

4. Breathe and look with the movement. Exhale as you pull your ribcage, looking left, and inhale as you release, allowing your spine (including your neck) to return to neutral.

5. Repeat on both sides.

➡ T-Spine rotation, grab rib cage and pull

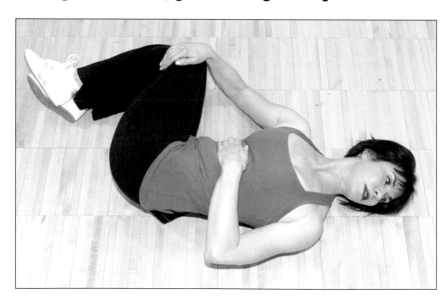

With an Arm Sweep
Key Points:

1. Extend your left arm flat on the floor and 90° to the side (straight off your shoulder).

2. With each inhale, sweep your arm up toward your ear as far as you can, while keeping your hand (palm up), wrist, elbow, and shoulder flat on the floor.

3. Exhale and return the arm to the starting position.

Note: The breathing during the arm-sweep version is reversed to expand your chest during the sweep overhead.

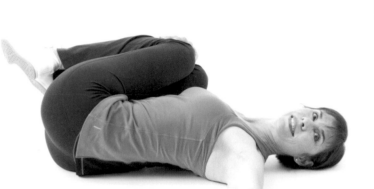

◯ Floor version: arm at 90°

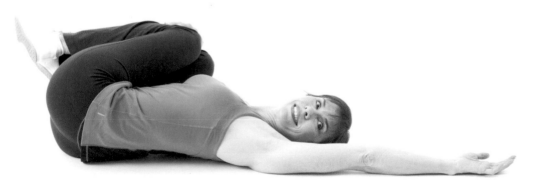

◯ Floor version: arm up by head

SEATED PUSH/PULL

Key Points:

1. Sit sideways on a chair that has a back.

2. Sit tall, with your right side facing the chair.

3. Make sure you are sitting on your "sits bones," keeping your knees together.

4. Grab hold of the back of the chair with both hands.

5. Use your hands to push/pull yourself into more rotation, getting as much rotation as you can without moving your hips or pelvis.

6. Exhale as you rotate, and inhale as you relax.

7. Stay tall. Do not slouch or round your lower back.

8. Repeat on both sides.

○ Seated version:
   Push/pul

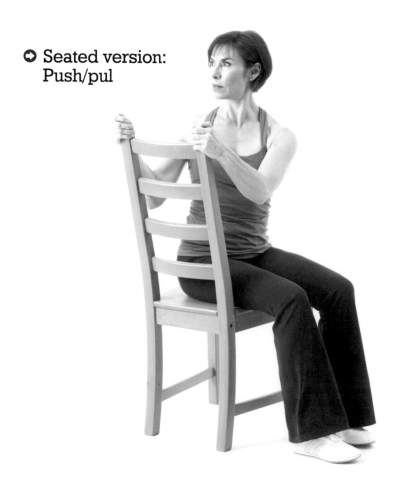

With an Arm Sweep
Key Points:

1. While rotating, extend your right arm and sweep it up.

2. Breathe in as your arm goes up and out as it goes down.

Note: The breathing with the arm sweep is reversed to expand your chest during the sweep overhead.

➲ Seated: arm at 90°

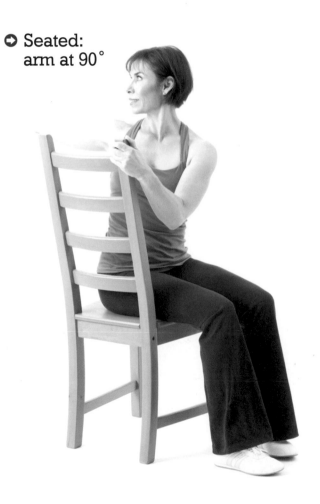

➲ Seated: arm up at head

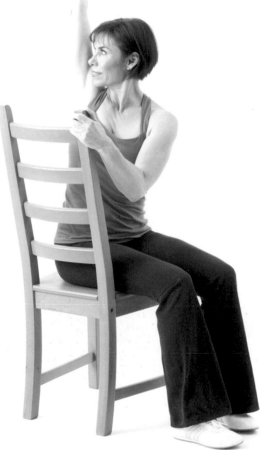

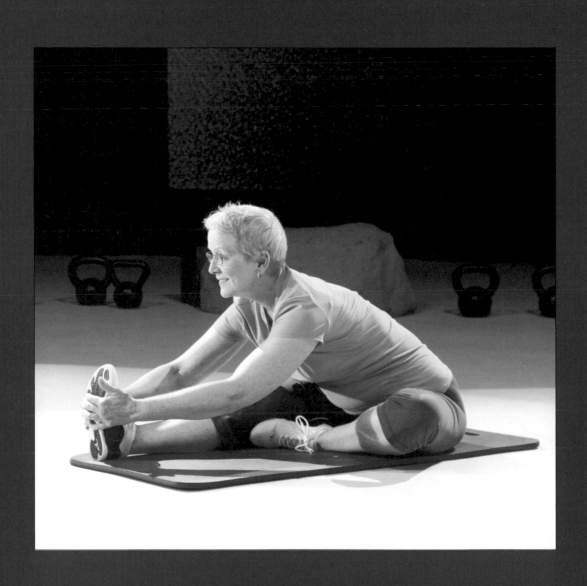

Chapter 6

Warm-Up Exercises

THREE-WAY NECK MOVEMENTS

Neck Rotation

Key Points:

1. Stand tall and press the top of your head to the ceiling.

2. Slowly rotate your head by turning your nose to the right in a smooth, slow movement. Then rotate left.

3. Go as far as you can go without forcing, and don't move into pain.

4. Keep your chin level. Don't let your chin move up or down at the end range of the movement.

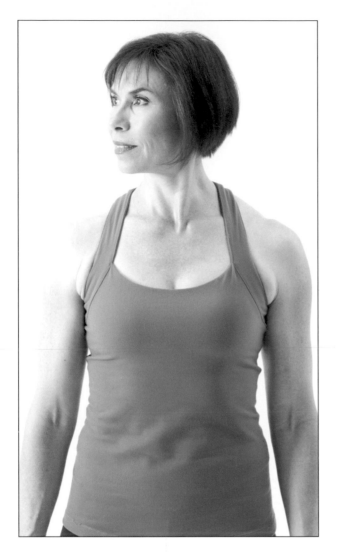 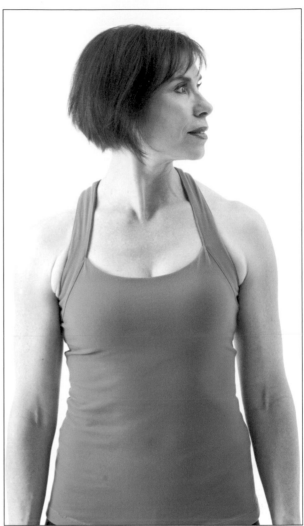

➲ Head rotate right

➲ Head rotate left

Neck Tilt
Key Points:

1. Tilt you your to the right, bringing your right ear to your shoulder

2. Imagine pressing your left ear and your jaw up to the ceiling.

3. Repeat on the other side.

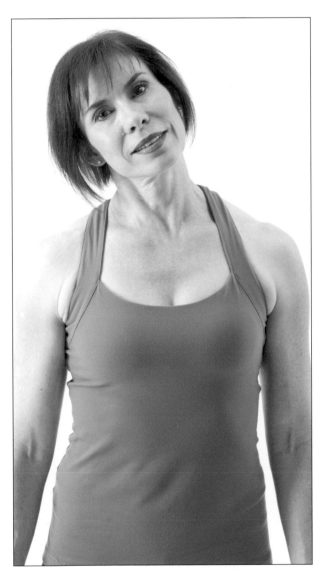

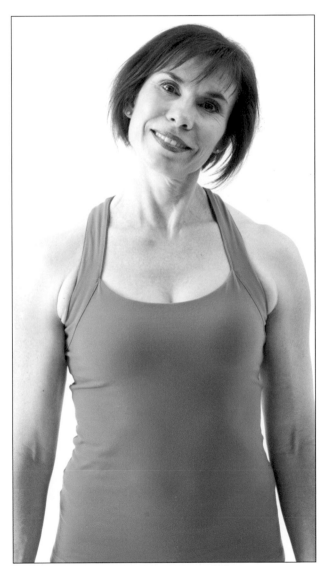

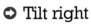 Tilt right   ➲ Tilt left

Chin Forward and Back
Key Points:

1. Push your chin forward.

2. Then push your chin as far back as possible.

3. Make sure to keep your chin level.

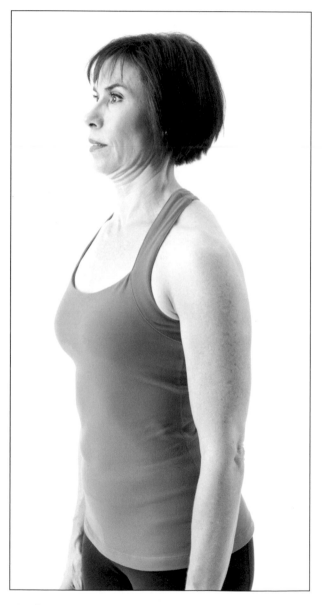

➲ Chin forward

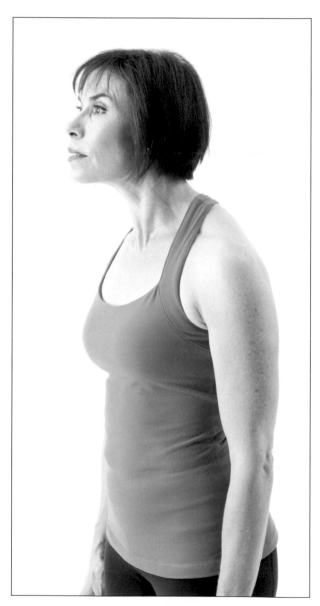

➲ Chin back

ARM AND SHOLUDER MOVEMENTS

Halo

Key Points:

1. Hold the kettlebell upside down by the "horns."

2. Slowly raise one elbow and begin to circle the kettlebell around your head.

3. Keep the kettlebell close to your chest and head during the movement.

4. Keep your biceps close to your head when your arms are in motion.

5. Keep your chest lifted and your chin level. Your head should not move to allow the kettlebell to pass.

6. Keep your glutes tight throughout the movement.

7. Gradually challenge the range of motion (how low the kettlebell dips behind you), as you go up in reps and become more comfortable with the exercise.

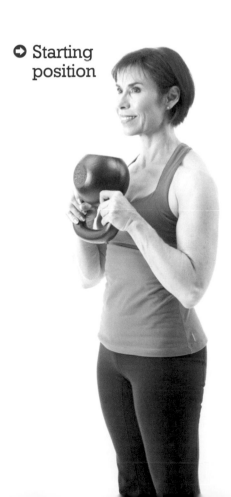

➲ Starting position

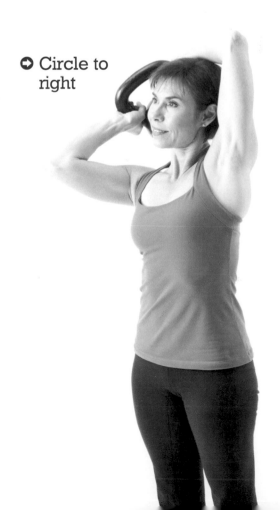

➲ Circle to right

⊙ Behind head   ⊙ Circle to left   ⊙ Ending

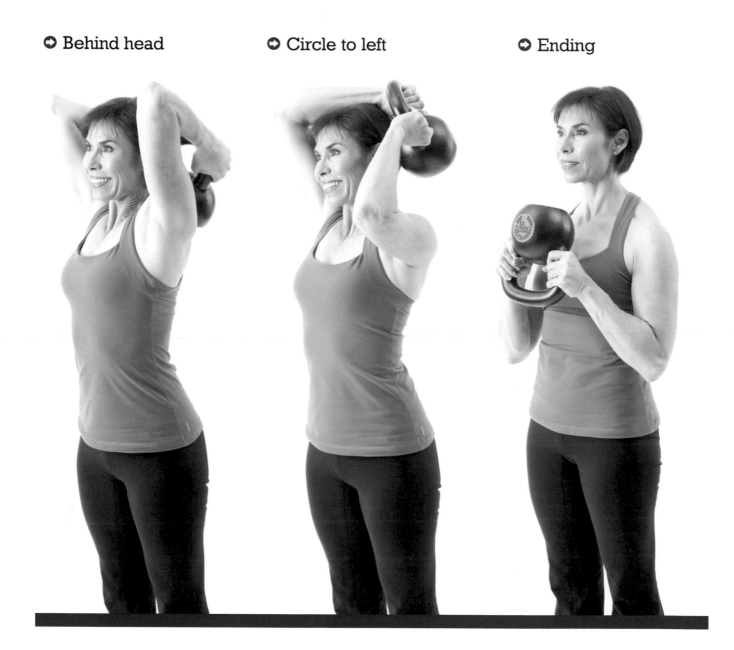

Note: Begin this drill by using your hands only, and then build up to using a kettlebell.

Shoulder Camshaft
Key Points:

1. Raise your arms to about shoulder height in front of you.

2. Lock out your elbows, and make fists.

3 .Start by reaching your arms forward and up. Then roll them back and down.

4. Create big, smooth, slow circles.

5. Feel your shoulder blades moving up and down, together and apart.

6. Repeat in the other direction.

➲ Shoulder Camshafts

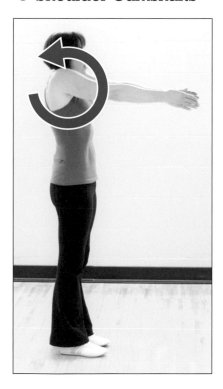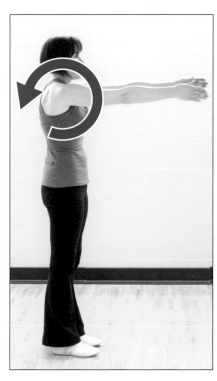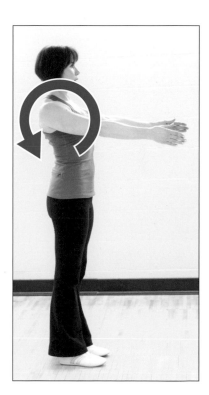

Egyptian
Key Points:

1. Raise your arms up and out to your sides, shoulder height.

2. Rotate to the right, drawing your right shoulder back and turning your palm up toward the ceiling.

3. Turn toward the hand that is rotating up by pivoting your feet and going onto the ball of your left foot.

4. As your right hand turns up, let your right elbow drop toward the floor.

5. Your left arm will rotate at the shoulder, pointing as far forward as it can. Corkscrew your left arm until your left palm is facing up.

6. Keep both arms up at shoulder height (especially your back arm).

7. Your torso may lean slightly in the direction you are facing.

8. Unwind this process and repeat it, turning to the left.

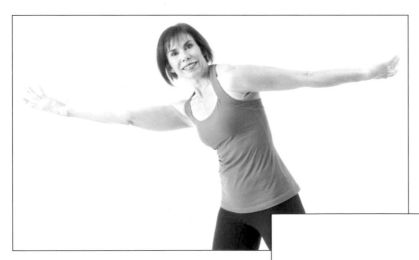

➲ Egyptian: Left

➲ Egyptian: Right

TORSO AND PELVIS MOVEMENTS

T-Spine

Key Points:

1. Stand tall, with your arms at your sides.

2 Inhale and make a big chest, lifting your sternum up and forward, as if being pulled up by a string.

3. Exhale and round out your upper back, as though your ribcage is being pulled behind you.

4. Your arms and shoulders will move a bit in this drill, but don't let them lead the movement.

5. Keep your arms, shoulders, and neck relaxed.

6. Keep your lower back and abs relaxed.

7. Repeat by inhaling and lifting your chest up and forward. Then exhale, sinking down, slumping slightly, and rounding your upper back.

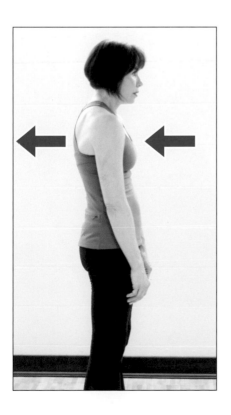 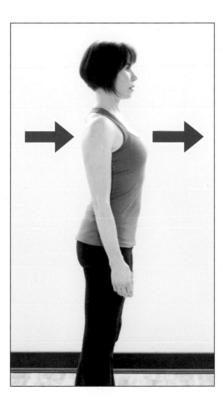

◒ T-Spine

Pelvis Circles
Key Points:

1. Stand with your feet hip distance apart and your feet pointing straight ahead.

2. Keep your knees slightly bent.

3. Rock or tilt your pelvis forward and backward.

4. Smoothly lift your pelvis side to side, as though you are lifting each hip bone up with a string.

5. Turn it into a full circle; imagine that you are using a hula-hoop. Repeat in both directions.

6. Your knees may move slightly with each movement.

➔ Front

➔ Back

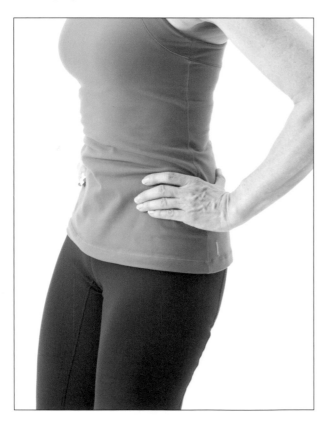 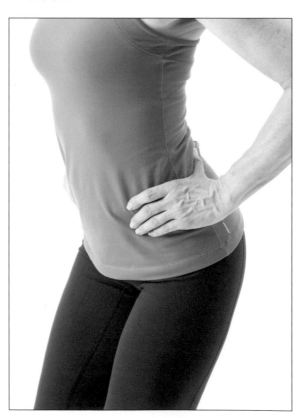

● Right side

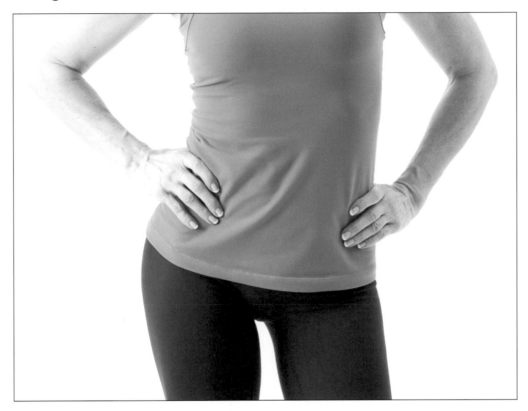

● Left side

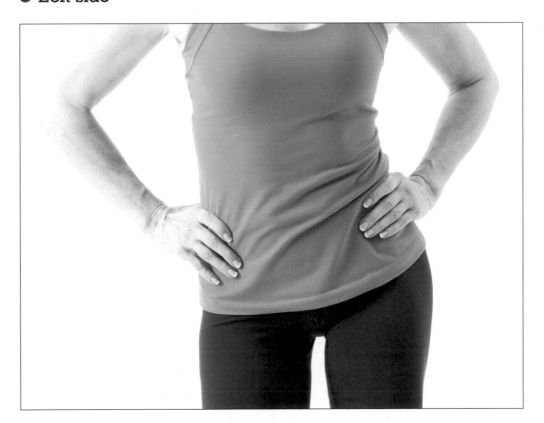

ELBOW, WRIST, AND FINGER MOVEMENTS

Elbow Circles

Key Points:

1. Lift your arms out in front of you, at shoulder height and about 45° from your body's midline.

2. Your arms should be parallel to the ground and mirroring each other.

3. Starting with your fists facing down, begin to circle your forearms toward your face.

4. Circle your fists over your shoulders, and keep circling them around until you lock out your elbows again in the starting position.

5. Rotate your palms down, and begin to form circles again.

6. Keep your elbows in the same place, and do not move from your shoulder.

7. Try not to let your upper arm rotate or move as you circle your lower arm.

8. Repeat in the opposite direction, bringing your arms around from outside to inside.

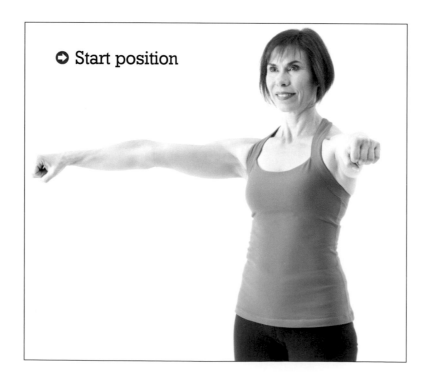

○ Start position

● Bend elbows

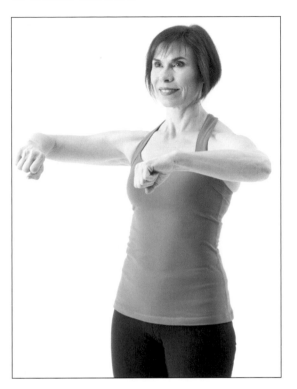

● Fist toward face

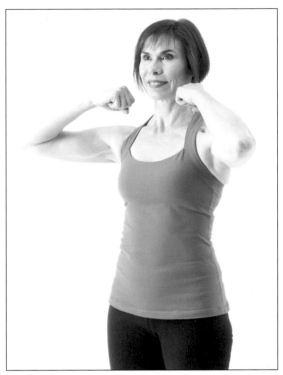

● Circle towards center

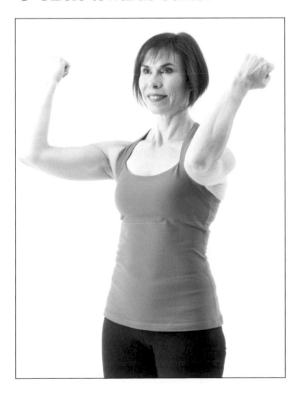

● Elbows lock out palm up

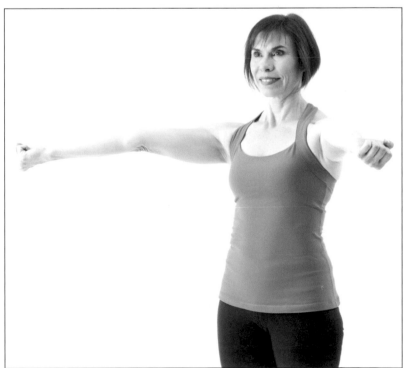

Wrist Mobility
Key Points:

1. Clasp your hands together at chest height.

2. Keeping your fingers locked together, gently circle your wrists around.

3. Repeat in the opposite direction.

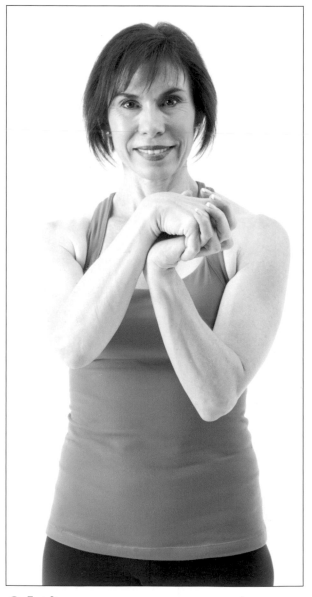

 Left

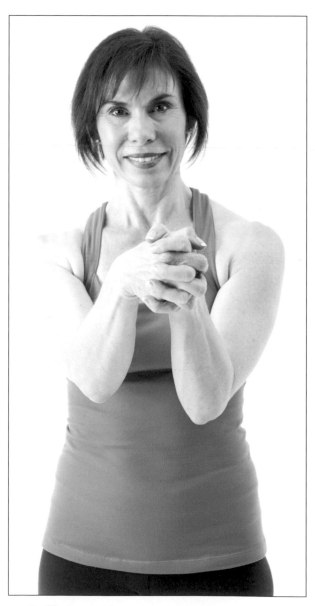

⊙ Forward

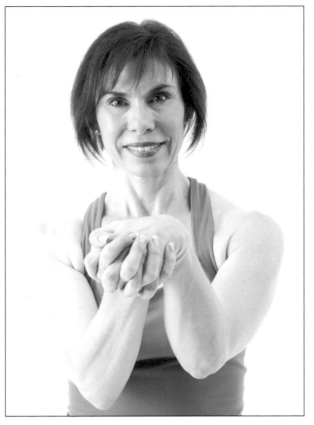

● Front

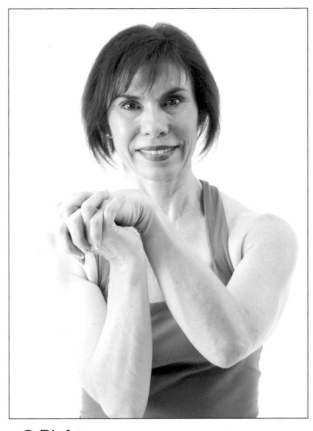

● Right

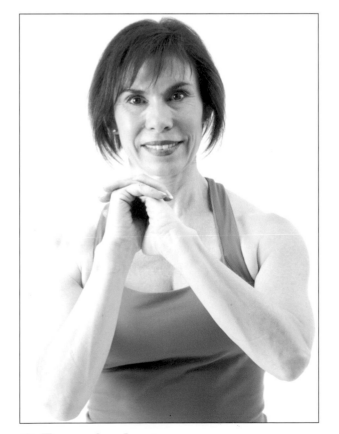

● Towards chest

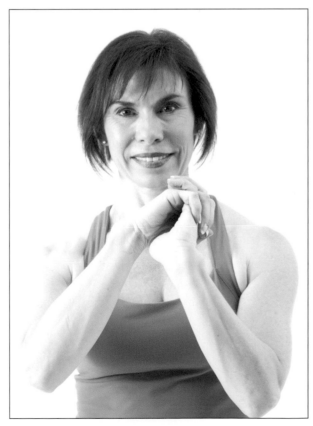

● Back towards left

Finger Mobility
Key Points:

1. Start with your fingers outstretched.

2. Starting from your fingertips, bend at each joint of your fingers and curl your hands into fists.

3. Pause and reverse the motion, beginning the movement from your knuckles and then restraightening your fingers one joint at a time.

4. Stretch out your fingers, making them as long as you can.

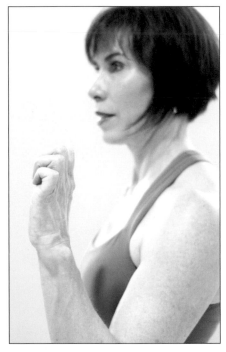
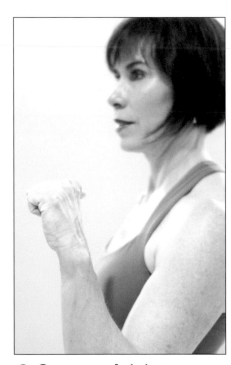
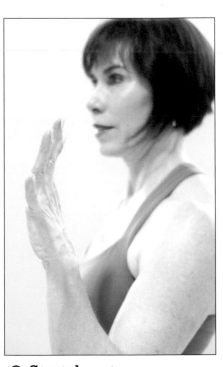

➲ Bend each joint   ➲ Open each joint   ➲ Stretch out

LEG AND FOOT MOVEMENTS
Leg Circles
Key Points:

1. Hold on to a chair at your left side for balance.

2. Shift your weight to your left leg, and stand tall and upright.

3. Lift your right leg out in front of you, high enough to clear the floor. Then circle it around to the side and back.

4. Keep your pelvis level and squared off to the front.

5. Keep your legs straight.

6. Repeat in the opposite direction, and then switch legs.

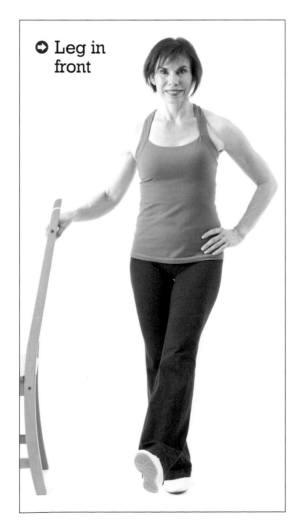

➲ Leg in front

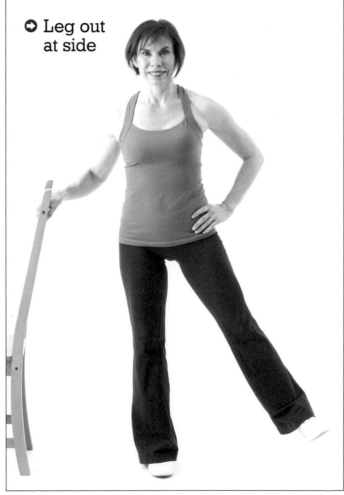

➲ Leg out at side

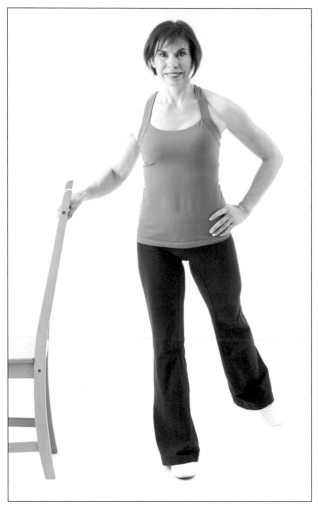

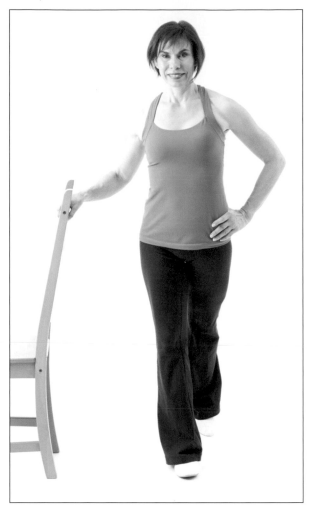

◐ Leg moves back

◐ Leg at back

Ankle Circles
Key Points:

1. Using a chair for balance, stand on one leg and extend the other out in front of you. (You can also sit tall in a chair and extend one leg out in front of you.)

2. Make big, slow circles with your ankle.

3. Try and make the movement as big and as smooth as possible, getting the full range of motion.

4. Repeat in the other direction.

5. Repeat on both sides.

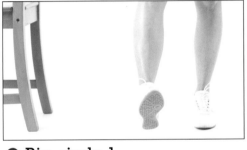

➲ Big circle 1

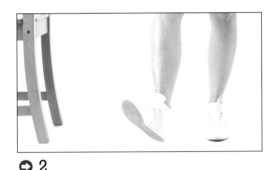

➲ 2

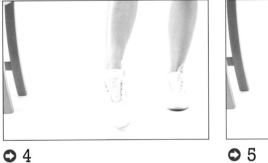

➲ 3

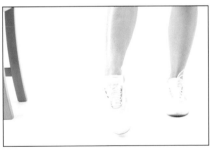

➲ 4

➲ 5

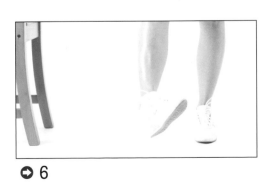

➲ 6

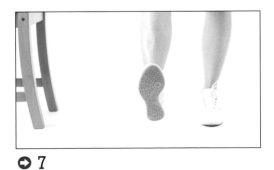

➲ 7

Foot Stretches
Key Points:

1. Holding on to a chair for balance, extend your right leg back and place the top of your foot on the floor directly behind you. (You may place a raised object—preferably something soft, like a rolled up towel—there to assist you in getting the top of your foot into the correct position.)

2. Slowly bend your supporting knee, and feel a gentle stretch on the top of your foot. Repeat this three times.

3. Drop your heel slightly to the outside, and gently stretch along the outside of your foot. Repeat this three times.

4. Perform both positions with both feet.

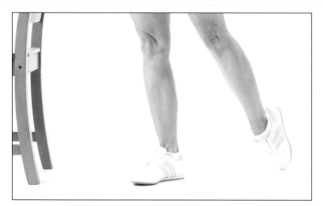

➡ Top of foot Stretch Start

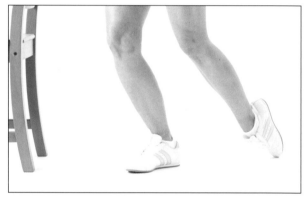

➡ Top of foot bend knee for stretch

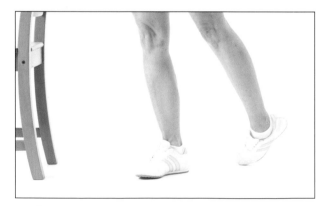

➡ Top of foot Stretch Start

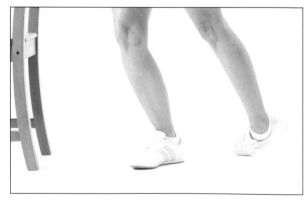

➡ Top of foot bend knee for stretch

Chapter 7

Main Kettlebell Exercises

DEADLIFT

With and without a Kettlebell

Key Points:

1. Stand with your feet hip distance apart.

2. Push your hips back, as you did in the hip hinge, with your arms either holding on to a chair (beginner) or reaching down between your legs to pick up the kettlebell.

3. Keep your eyes looking straight ahead or slightly down.

4. Keep your lats and upper back engaged. Do not let your shoulders roll forward or shrug up toward your ears.

5. Keep your weight on your heels and your shins as vertical as possible.

6. Your knees should be tracking your toes and should not bend so much that they reach out beyond them.

7. If you are using a kettlebell, brace your abdominals before you stand up.

8. Press your feet hard into the ground, and lengthen your spine as you stand up.

9. At the top, squeeze your glutes as hard as possible while you pull up your kneecaps.

10. Your body should now form a straight line through your ankles, knees, hips, back, shoulders, and head.

> **Note:** If your Self-Screen indicated that you have limited hip mobility, use a platform that raises the kettlebell up to the height that allows you to maintain proper back alignment. This is especially important if you have had a hip or knee replacement or injury.

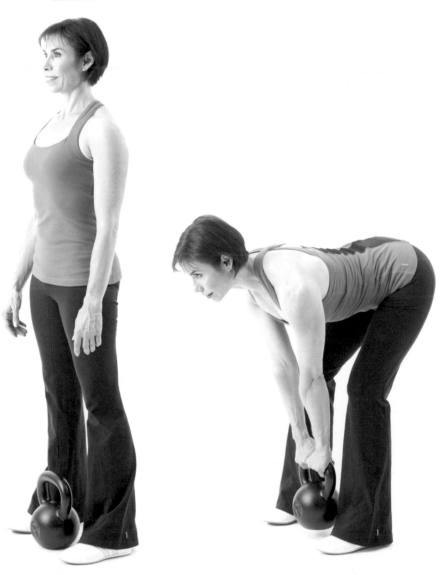

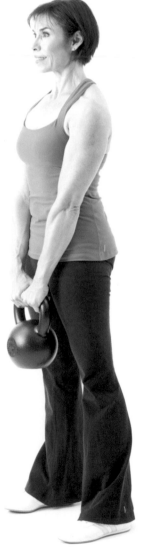

⊙ Standing with KB between feet (1-Int/Adv)

⊙ Bending over grabbing KB (2-Int/Adv)

⊙ Standing up straight (3-Int/Adv)

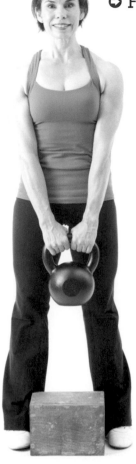

➲ From box (1-Beg)

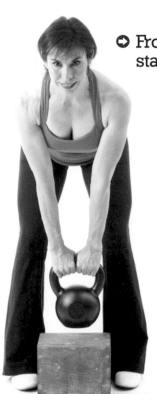

➲ From box
standing up (2-Beg)

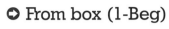

- **DO NOT** at any point let your knees push forward of your toes.

- **DO NOT** at any time let your lower back round (see neutral pelvis).

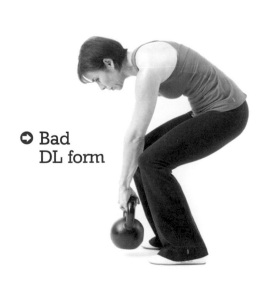

➲ Bad
DL form

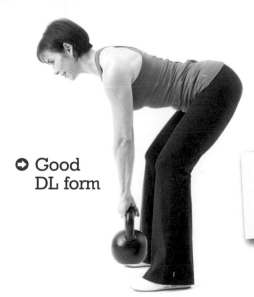

➲ Good
DL form

Note: Here is
what it should
look like.

Suitcase Deadlift
Key Points:

1. Stand in a deadlift position but this time, with the kettlebell on your right side, next to your foot.

2. Start pushing your hips back, as in the regular deadlift.

3. Keep your shoulders and hips perfectly level, and reach down and grip the kettlebell with your right hand. It helps to imagine that you are reaching for a second kettlebell with your left hand.

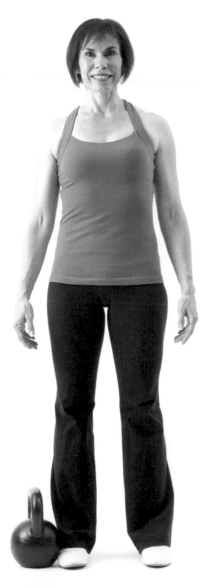

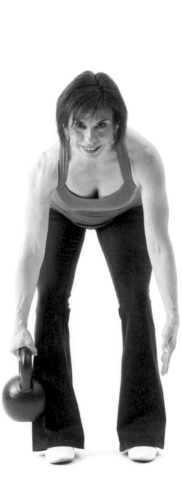

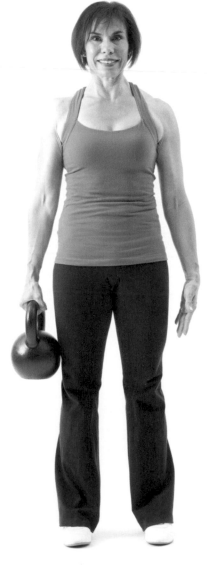

➲ KB at side –
   standing (1 - Int/Adv)

➲ Picking KB up
   (2 - Int/Adv)

➲ Standing up
   with KB (3 - Int/Adv)

4. Make sure to keep your lats engaged, and do not allow your shoulders to roll forward.

5. Keeping your elbow straight and your knees tracking your toes, sniff in some air, bracing with your abs and obliques, and pick up the kettlebell from the ground.

6. Stand up, keeping your shoulders in a straight line.

7. Squeeze your glutes as hard as possible, while keeping your abdominals tight. Get tall to finish.

8. All other points apply for performing the deadlift.

9. Repeat on the other side.

Note: Use a platform if necessary.

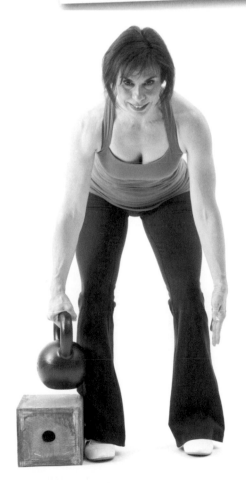

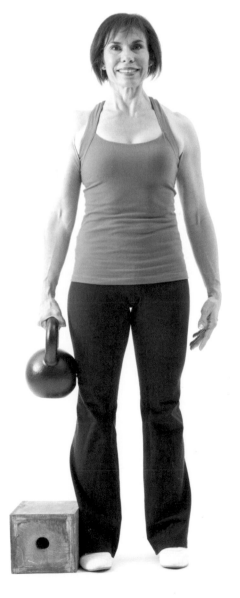

➲ KB on box (1 - Beg)

➲ KB on box picking kb up (2 - Beg)

Suitcase Deadlift
Key Points:

1. Stand as in the suitcase deadlift position, the kettlebell next to your foot.

2. Stand tall on the leg nearest the kettlebell, while the other leg reaches back. You may at any time place that foot on the ground for balance.

3. Start pushing your butt back, as in the hinge. Keep your abs tight and your spine neutral.

4. Keep your shoulders and hips perfectly level as you reach down and pick up the kettlebell with one arm. It helps to imagine that you are reaching for a second kettlebell with your other hand.

5. All other points apply for performing the deadlift.

6. Repeat on the other side.

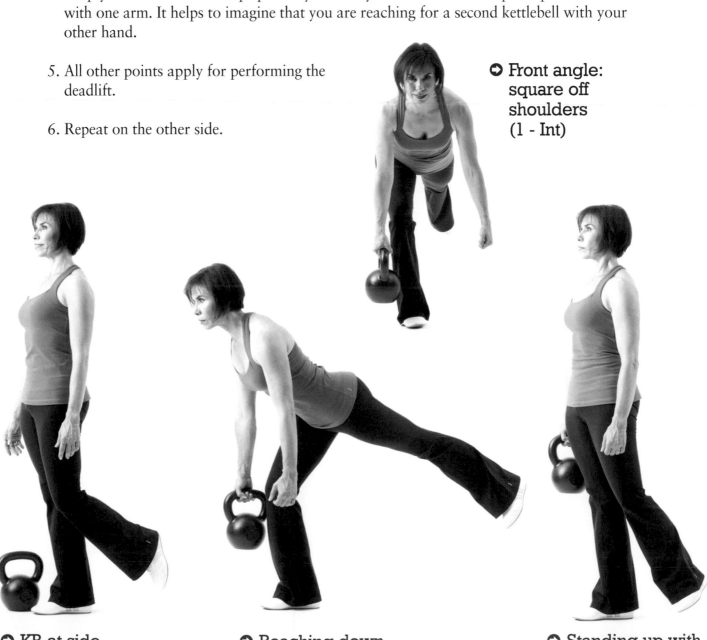

➲ Front angle:
square off
shoulders
(1 - Int)

➲ KB at side –
standing (1 - Int/Adv)

➲ Reaching down
for KB (2 - Int)

➲ Standing up with
KB (3 - Int)

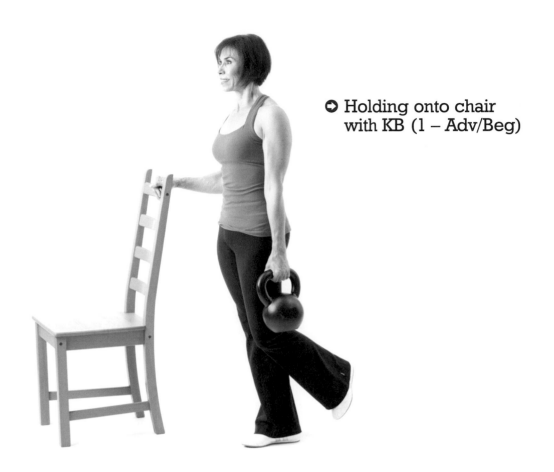

⊙ Holding onto chair
with KB (1 – Adv/Beg)

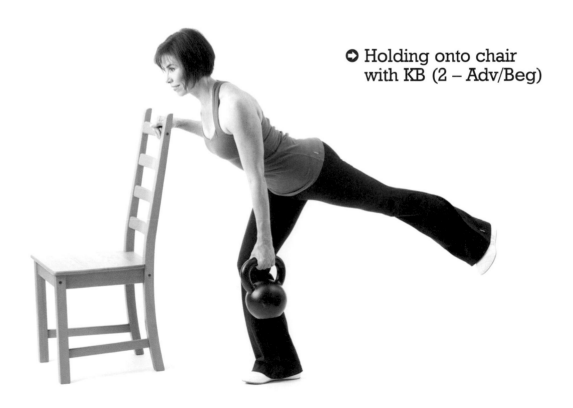

⊙ Holding onto chair
with KB (2 – Adv/Beg)

○ Hold chair
  without KB (1 - Beg)

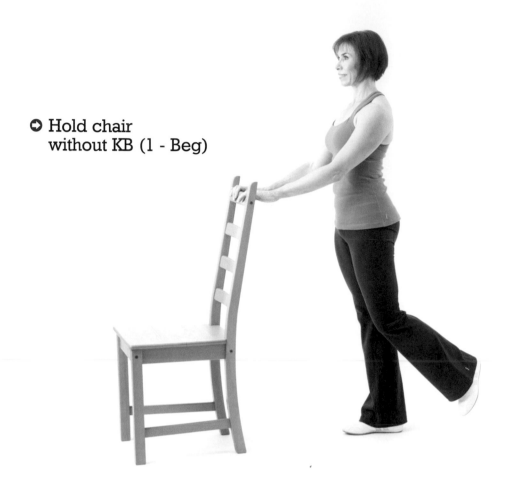

○ Holding chair
  without KB (2 - Beg)

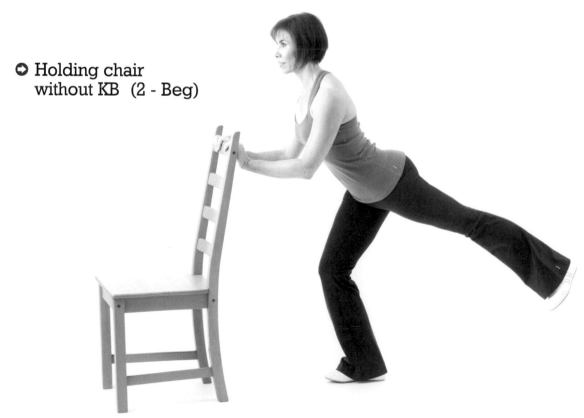

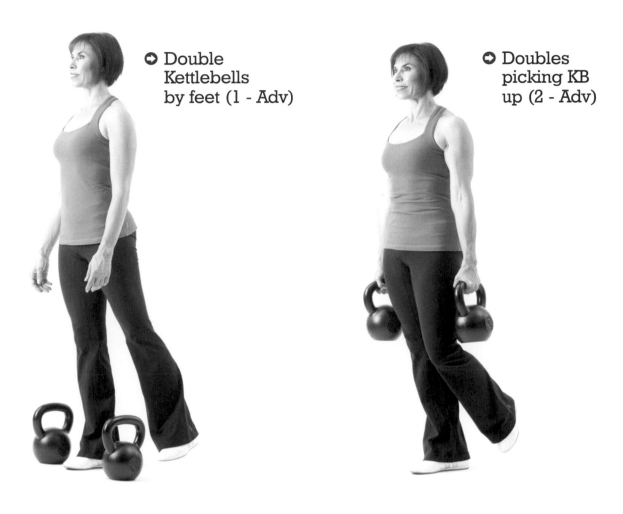

➲ Double
  Kettlebells
  by feet (1 - Adv)

➲ Doubles
  picking KB
  up (2 - Adv)

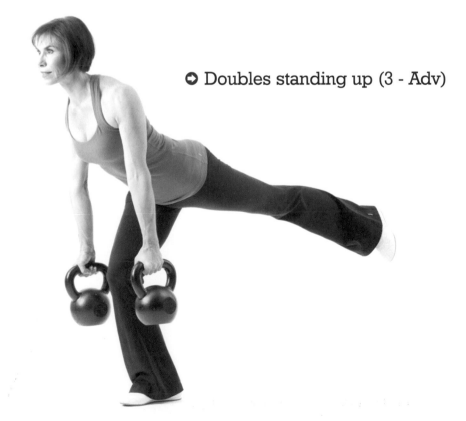

➲ Doubles standing up (3 - Adv)

CARRY

Kettlebell carries strengthen the shoulders, back, and core. Performing them is a fast way to achieve good posture and healthy shoulders.

Farmer's Walk
Key Points:

1. Start by performing a suitcase deadlift.

2. Lift the shoulder of your working arm up and roll it down and back to feel a squeeze in your armpit. (If you are using two kettlebells, pinch your shoulder blades together.)

3. Keep your chest lifted, your chin level, and your elbow locked.

4. Do not allow your shoulder to drop.

5. Carefully set the kettlebell down with a suitcase deadlift movement.

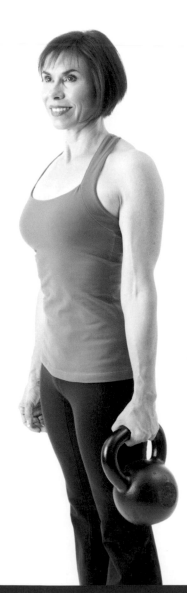

◗ Holding KB at side (1 - Beg)

Clean Position
Key Points:

1. Clean or cheat curl the kettlebell up to the clean position. Make sure that the bell portion of the kettlebell is placed equally between your bicep and forearm.

2. Your wrist MUST remain straight, and you MUST try to keep your forearm as vertical as possible.

3. Actively squeeze your arm against your ribcage, and let your shoulder sink down.

4. Ladies, make sure you are not pressing your arm against your breast. Instead, pull your arm in, against your ribcage.

5. Squeeze and tighten your lat, chest, bicep, and abdominal muscles as you walk.

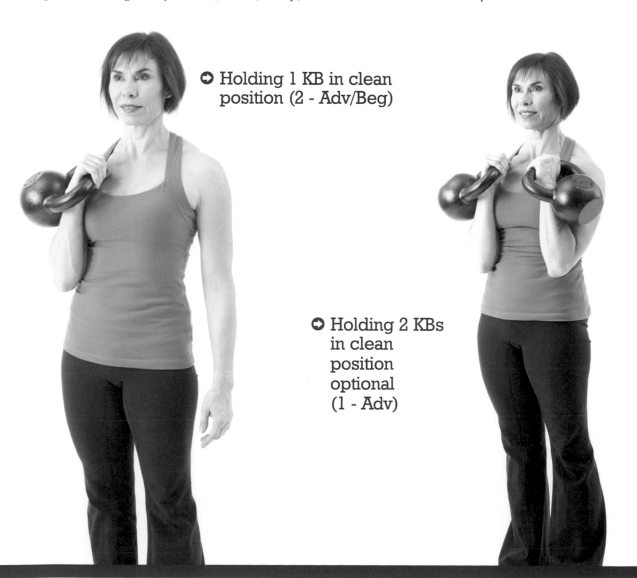

➲ Holding 1 KB in clean position (2 - Adv/Beg)

➲ Holding 2 KBs in clean position optional (1 - Adv)

Waiter's Walk
Key Points:

1. Press the kettellbell overhead.

2. Keep your shoulder down and packed.

3. Your elbow should remain locked.

4. Your wrist must remain straight.

5. All other points apply for performing the military press.

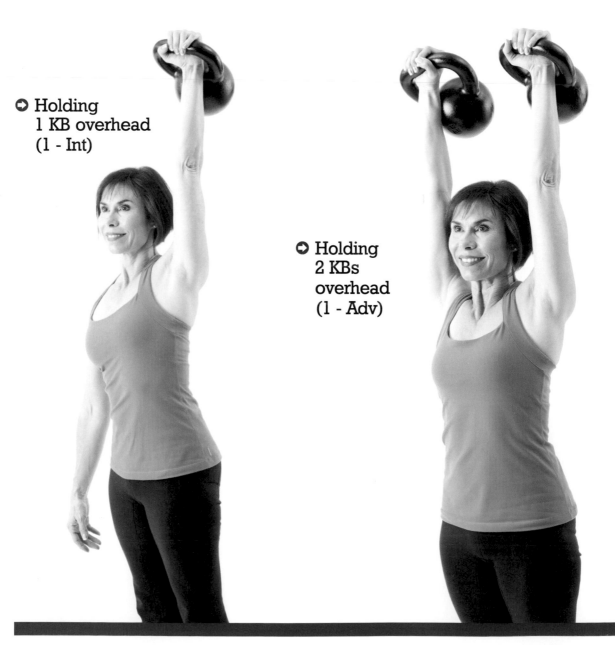

○ Holding
   1 KB overhead
   (1 - Int)

○ Holding
   2 KBs
   overhead
   (1 - Adv)

PLANK
From Elbows and Feet
Key Points:

1. Lay face down, pressed up onto your elbows and toes.

2. Your body should form a straight line from the top of your head to your heels.

3. Imagine that you are bringing together your tailbone and your belly button.

4. Flatten your lower back. Do not let it dip down.

5. Squeeze your glutes tight.

6. Pull up your kneecaps, and tighten your quads.

7. Tighten your lats by pulling your elbows and shoulders down, toward your waist.

8. Look straight down.

9. Breathe shallowly into a tight stomach.

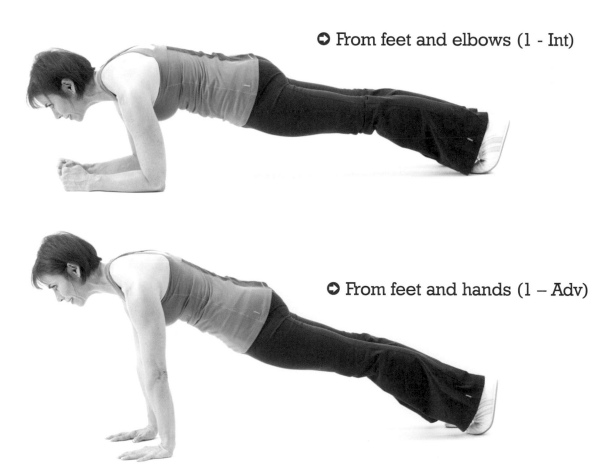

➲ From feet and elbows (1 - Int)

➲ From feet and hands (1 – Adv)

From Elbows and Knees
Key Points:

1. Lay face down, pressed up onto your elbows and knees. (Make sure that your knees are well padded.)

2. Your body should form a straight line from the top of your head to your knees.

3. Imagine that you are bringing together your tailbone and your belly button.

4. Flatten your lower back. Do not let it dip down.

5. Squeeze your glutes tight.

6. Tighten your lats by pulling your elbows and shoulders down, toward your waist.

7. Look straight down.

8. Breathe shallowly into a tight stomach.

➔ From knees and elbows (1 - Adv/Beg)

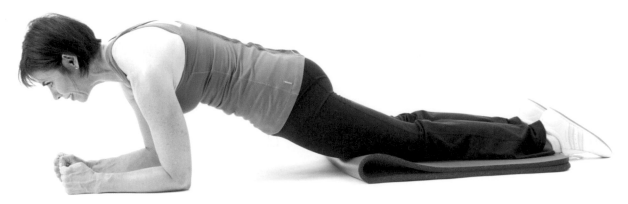

Elbows on the Wall
Key Points:

1. Stand about 1 foot from a wall.

2. Place your elbows on the wall at shoulder height.

3. Lean against the wall with your elbows, adjusting your feet so that as much of your weight as possible is on your elbows.

4. Your body should form a straight line from the top of your head to your knees.

5. Imagine that you are bringing together your tailbone and your belly button.

6. Flatten your lower back. Do not let it dip down.

7. Squeeze your glutes tight.

8. Pull up your kneecaps, and tighten your quads.

9. Tighten your lats by pulling your elbows and shoulders down, toward your waist.

10. Look straight out to the wall.

11. Breathe shallowly into a tight stomach.

12. You can either lift up your heels or keep them flat on the floor. This drill isn't a calf stretch, so you can raise your heels if you feel too much of a stretch in your lower leg.

Note: Start with your feet closer to the wall, as you develop strength move your feet further away from the wall.

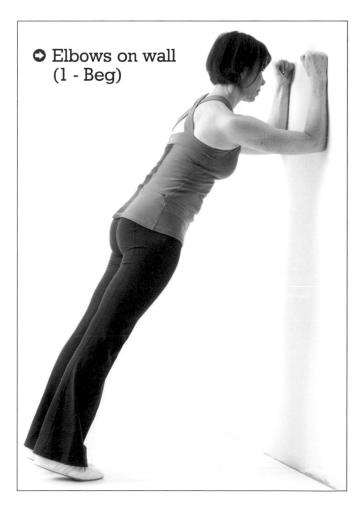

○ Elbows on wall
(1 - Beg)

SWING

The swing is an important tool for creating a strong, healthy back and powerful hips. It is a very athletic movement that can benefit anyone who is able to perform it safely.

Key Points:

1. Your hips and lower body must follow a deadlift pattern, NOT a squat pattern.

2. Your shins should remain as vertical as possible, with little to no forward movement of the knees.

3. Your back must remain straight or neutral throughout the movement.

4. Reach back with your hips, not down. (Reaching down encourages the shins to break vertical.)

5. Hike the kettlebell between your legs and toward your tailbone.

6. Keep your heels down, pressing your feet strongly into the floor.

7. Your knees must track your toes. Your feet may turn out SLIGHTLY but not more than 45°.

8. Snap your hips forward aggressively from the bottom of the movement, and extend your hips fully at the top by forcefully clamping your glutes together.

9. Your body should achieve a straight line at the top. Do not let your upper body lean back. Instead, flex your abs and think of getting tall.

10. Pull your kneecaps up to tighten your quads. DO NOT force your knees back.

11. Keep your arms straight and your shoulders down throughout the movement. Think of the kettlebell as an extension of your loose arms. It should not flip upward.

12. Use biomechanical breathing. Inhale sharply and tighten your abs during the backswing, and exhale sharply as your hips extend—not when the kettlebell reaches the top.

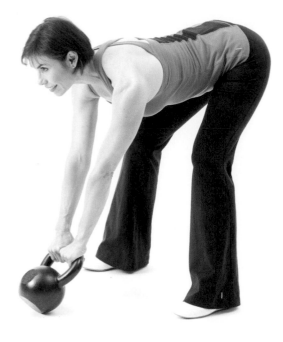

➲ 2-hand bottom-start position (1 - Beg)

➲ 2-hand hike position (2 - Beg)

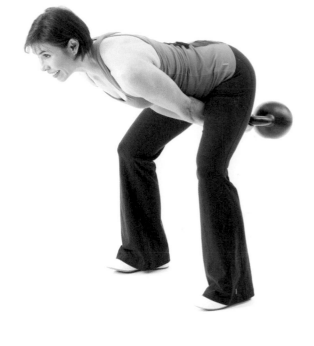

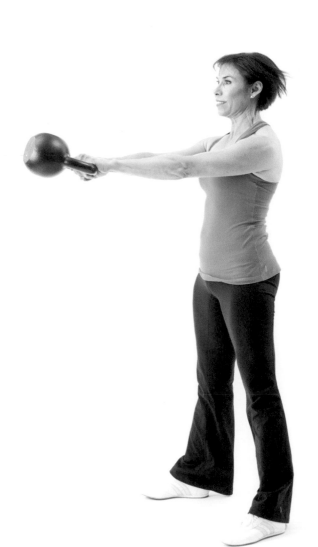

➲ 2-hand top position (3 - Beg)

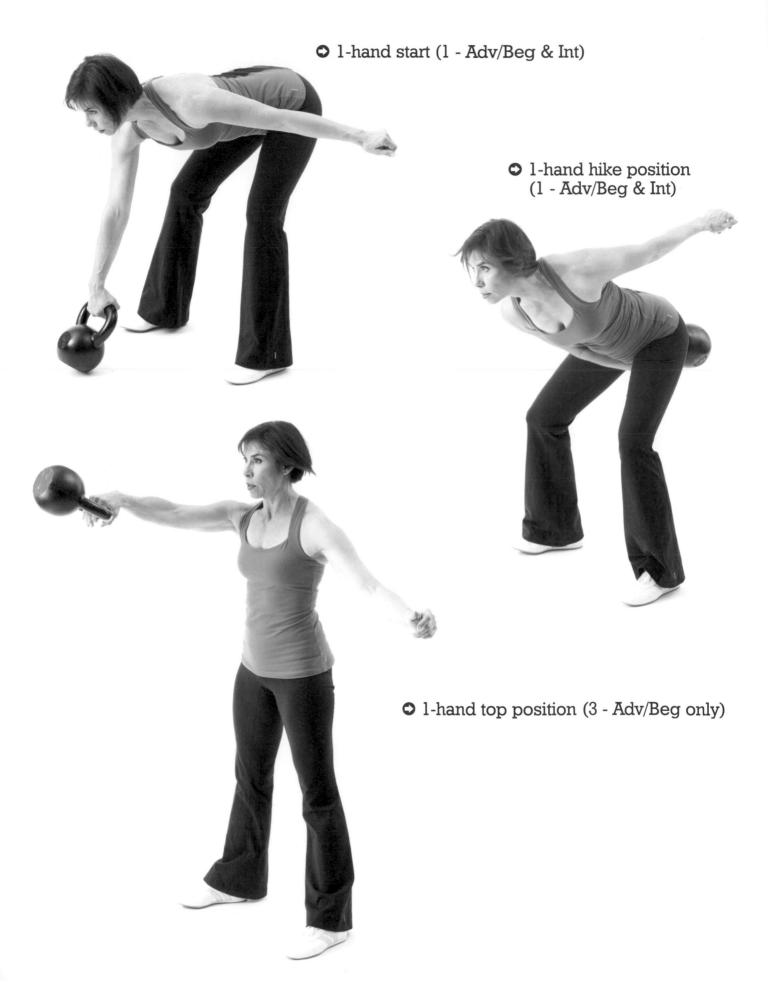

➲ 1-hand start (1 - Adv/Beg & Int)

➲ 1-hand hike position
(1 - Adv/Beg & Int)

➲ 1-hand top position (3 - Adv/Beg only)

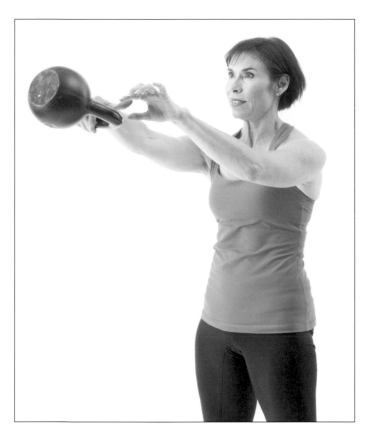

➡ Hand to hand switch
(3 - Int *only*)

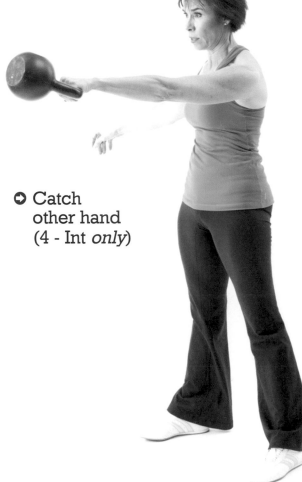

➡ Catch
other hand
(4 - Int *only*)

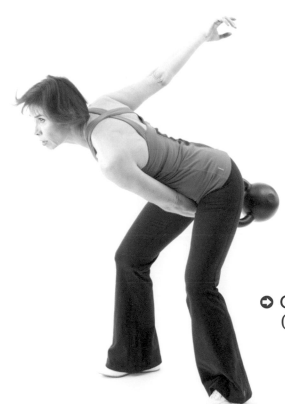

➡ Opposite hand, bottom position
(5 - Int *only*)

PRESS

The benefits of performing the RKC press are the emphasis on healthy shoulder movement and the technique that supports it. It is a great drill in full-body tension and is a favorite for developing upper-body strength and coordination.

Key Points:

1. Clean or cheat curl the kettlebell into the rack position. Pause, keeping your body tight.

2. Start to press with your fist at collarbone level, your kneecaps pulled up, your glutes squeezed tight, and your abs engaged.

3. Keep your forearm vertical throughout the movement.

◆ Standing clean position
(1 - Adv/Beg)

◆ Standing start press
(2 - Adv/Beg)

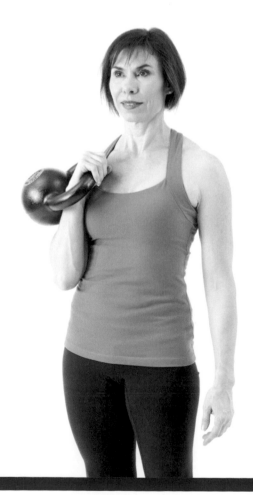

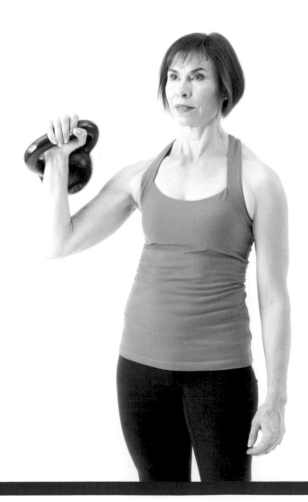

4. Keep your shoulders down. Do not let them shrug up, toward your ears.

5. Lock out your elbow to finish at the top. Your arm should be near your ear and your shoulder packed.

6. Power breathe. DO NOT exhale completely during the press. You may inhale slightly at the top and then hiss out more air on the descent.

7. When lowering the kettlebell, keep your body tight and grounded. You may slowly pull the kettlebell toward you, as if you are doing a chin-up (advanced), or simply control its descent.

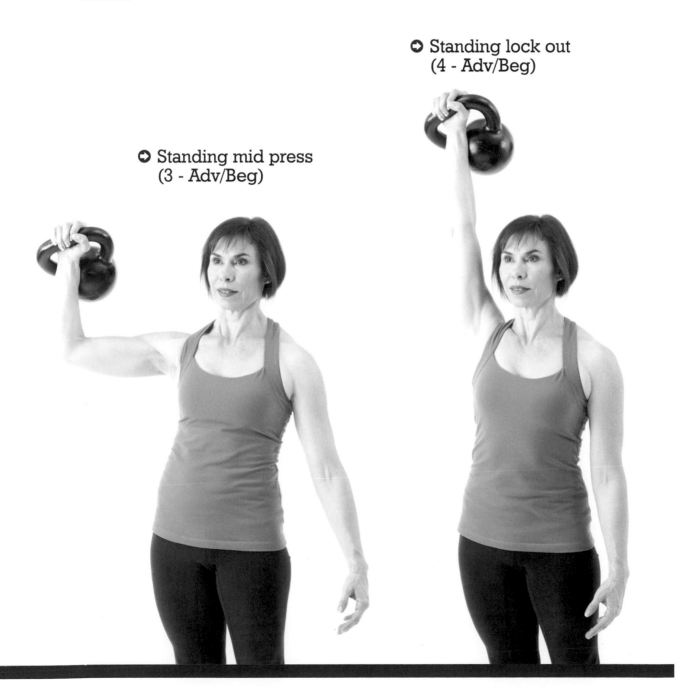

◆ Standing lock out (4 - Adv/Beg)

◆ Standing mid press (3 - Adv/Beg)

Seated Assisted Version
Key Points:

1. Sit tall on your "sits bones."

2. Start in the clean position, but have your assisting hand grab on top of your working hand.

3. The kettlebell needs to track slightly in front of you. You will not be able to open your pressing arm out to the side.

4. Once you have locked out the press, tighten your lats and pull the kettlebell down. If possible, release your assisting arm and let your working arm bring the kettlebell back down into the rack position.

5. All other points apply for performing the press.

⊃ Seated-assisted top (3 - Beg)

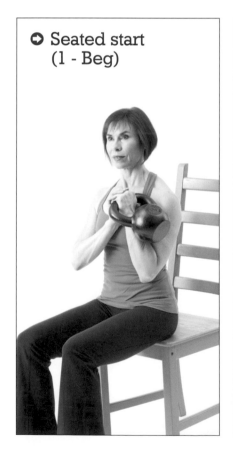

⊃ Seated start (1 - Beg)

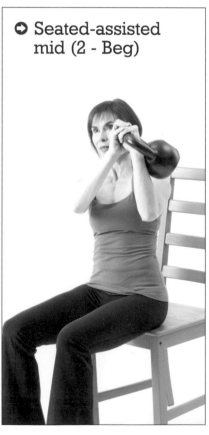

⊃ Seated-assisted mid (2 - Beg)

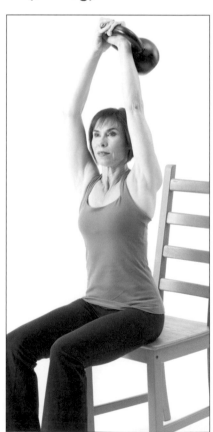

Kneeling On Floor
Key Points:

1. Kneel on a padded surface, knees hip distance apart.

2. Push your pelvis forward and squeeze your glutes tight.

3. Keep your abdominals tight throughout the press.

4. All other points apply for performing the press.

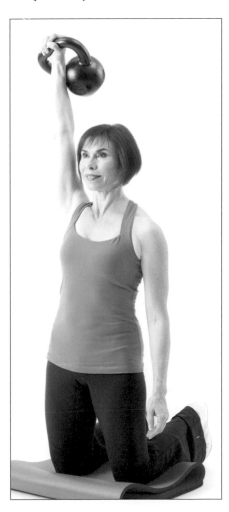

➲ Kneeling lock out
(3 - Int)

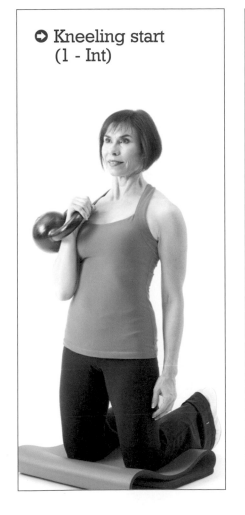

➲ Kneeling start
(1 - Int)

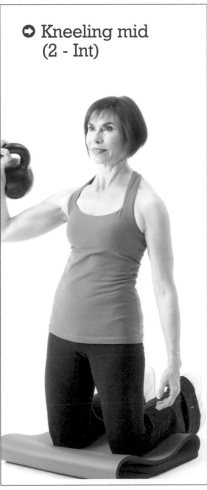

➲ Kneeling mid
(2 - Int)

One-Legged or with One Leg on a Box
Key Points:

1. Pull up your kneecaps, and squeeze your glutes as hard as possible.

2. Feel your foot firmly planted on the floor, and stand tall.

3. Keep your abdominals and obliques very tight as the kettlebell moves slightly out toward the side, following the same groove as the other presses.

4. If you are using a box for your nonweighted foot, make sure you place little or none of your weight on the box.

5. If you are not using a box, you can lift your leg in front or hold it behind you.

6. All other points apply for performing the standing press.

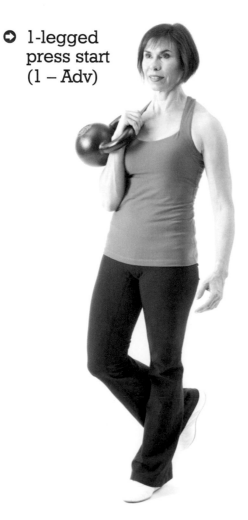

⟳ 1-legged
press start
(1 – Adv)

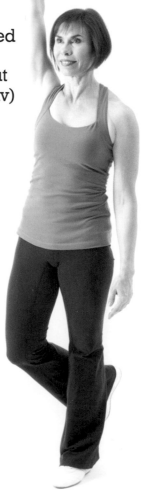

⟳ 1-legged
press
lock out
(2 – Adv)

GOBLET SQUAT

The goblet squat is an excellent leg strengthener, and it has the added bonus of developing hip flexibility. EVERYONE can squat. You just need to learn the safe, proper technique.

Key Points:

1. Find your squat stance, with your feet slightly wider than shoulder width apart. Remember that your stance may be narrower than you think. Your feet should point as close to straight ahead as possible.

2. Hold the kettlebell by the "horns." Keeping your chest lifted, bend at the knees and start pushing your butt back.

3. Keeping your back straight, try and push your knees out. You should feel as though you are pulling yourself down as you go.

4. At the bottom, your elbows should rest on the insides of your knees (the vastus medialis) or thighs. Push your elbows out, against your knees.

5. Keep your spine tall and straight. Never squat to a depth where you can no longer maintain a straight back.

6. Grunt as you start to come up. Make sure that your head and chest lead your hips. Do not allow your heels or big toes to come off the ground.

7. Finish at the top with a glute squeeze, your kneecaps pulled up, as in the top of the swing.

➡ Box Squat holding chair
start (1 - Beg)

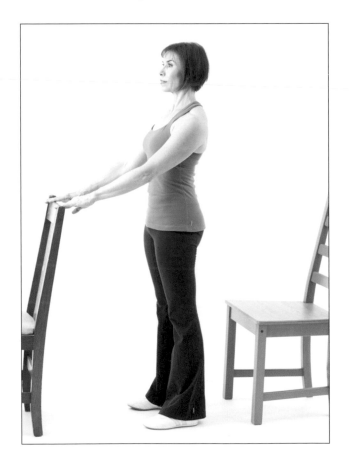

➡ Box Squat holding chair
end (2 - Beg)

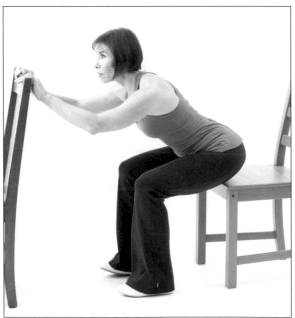

⭕ Box Squat KB & Chair
start (1 - Adv/Beg)

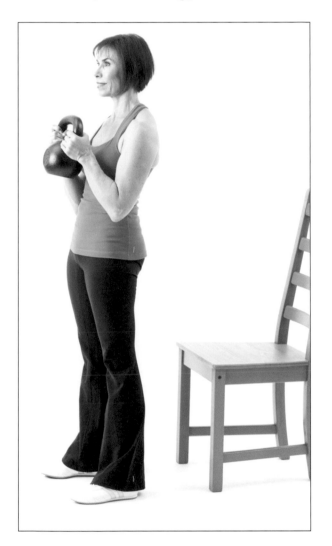

⭕ Box Squat KB & Chair
end (2 -Adv/Beg)

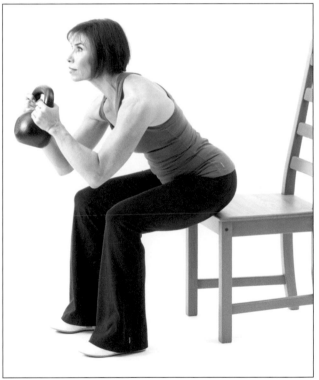

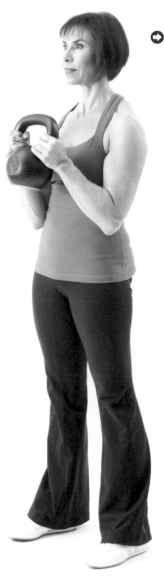

➡ Goblet start (1 - Int)

➡ Goblet end (2 - Int)

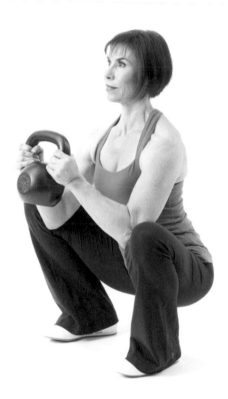

RUSSIAN TWISTS

Seated in a Chair
(with or without a kettlebell)

Key Points:

1. Sit tall in a chair, with your feet and knees together.

2. Hold the kettlebell by the horns.

3. Inhale. Then exhale and rotate slightly to the right, squeezing your abs and obliques.

4. Keep your "sits bones" firmly on the chair.

5. You can add a slight crunch at the end of the rotation.

6. Inhale and then exhale as you work the opposite direction.

7. Do not slouch. Get tall between reps.

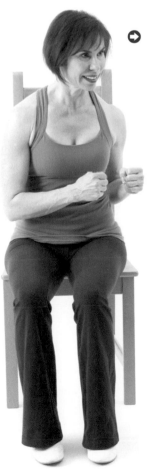

➲ On Chair
no KB (1 - Beg)

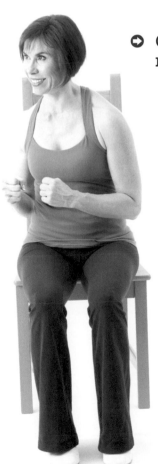

➲ On Chair
no KB (2 - Beg)

● On Chair
   with KB (1 - Beg)

● On Chair
   with KB (2 - Beg)

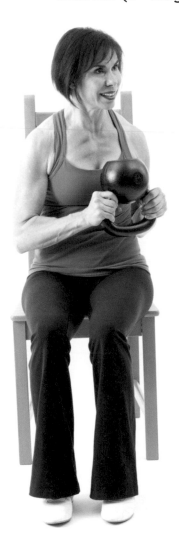

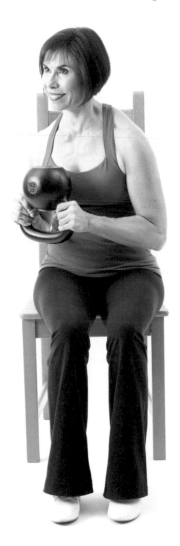

Standing
Key Points:

1. Stand with your feet close together.

2. Hold the kettlebell by the horns, keeping your glutes tight.

3. Inhale. Then exhale and rotate slightly to the right, squeezing your abs and obliques.

4. You can add a slight crunch at the end of the rotation.

5. Inhale and then exhale as you work the opposite direction. You may crunch slightly over the leg that you are turning toward, but make sure to keep your glutes tight.

6. Once again, get tall between reps.

⊙ Standing (1 - Int)   ⊙ Standing (2 - Int)

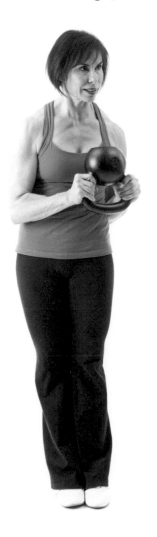   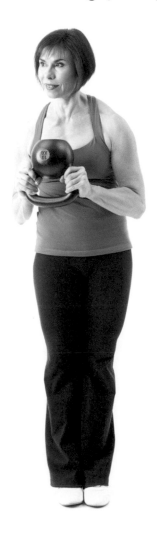

Seated on the Floor
Key Points:

1. Sit back to form a V shape with your torso and thighs. Keep your knees bent.

2. Your weight should be slightly behind your "sits bones," and your lower back should be flexed.

3. Inhale. Then exhale and rotate to the right. Your knees may lean away from the crunch.

4. You may lift your feet off of the floor to make the exercise more difficult.

5. Inhale and then exhale as you work the opposite direction.

6. Keep your abs tight for the duration of the exercise.

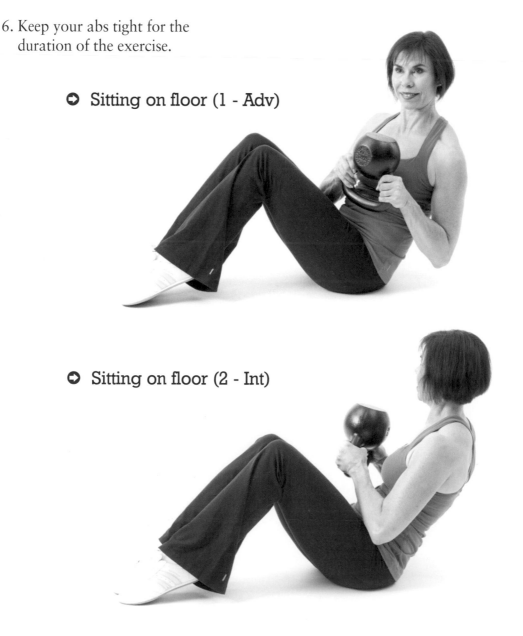

➲ **Sitting on floor (1 - Adv)**

➲ **Sitting on floor (2 - Int)**

Chapter 8

The Get-Up

The get-up is an important exercise for shoulder stability, mobility, and strength. It requires you to keep your core firing and your shoulder stable while you move your body from a supine to a standing position.

Start using no weight or holding on to a shoe or a water bottle. Move on to holding a kettlebell only when you have learned the movement pattern thoroughly and developed enough strength to hold a kettlebell overhead (as described in the Carry section in Chapter 7).

Key Points:

1. Lying on your back, roll on to your right side. Grab the kettlebell with your right hand, using your left hand to assist your right. Pull and roll on to your back, with the bell portion against your arm. Both arms should rest against your chest. Also, your shoulders must remain packed down and your lats engaged for the remainder of the exercise.

2. Press the kettlebell overhead with both hands. Your eyes cannot leave the kettlebell until you reach the kneeling position. Once your right elbow is locked above your chest, lower your left arm to the ground so that it is 45° from your side, palm down. Bend your right knee and place your foot 45° from your body, foot flat. Your right foot should not need to move from this position and will remain flat at all times. Again, keep your *shoulder pressed down* and your lat engaged. Your *elbow remains locked* throughout the drill, and your *wrist remains straight*.

3. Using the elbow of your left arm and your right foot, turn your hips and roll slightly to your left and up onto your left forearm. Note that now, your left shoulder is engaged and must be pressed down into the socket. Push your chest out and slightly up. Reaching with your left heel will prevent your left leg from lifting up during this phase. This sit-up to (and down from) the elbow portion of the exercise is the only segment in which the arm holding the kettlebell is allowed to lean forward slightly to aid you.

4. Sit up until you are supporting yourself with your left hand, and "screw" your supporting shoulder into the socket. Keep your neck elongated and both shoulders packed down.

5. Pushing your left hand and your FLAT right foot into the ground, lift your hips slightly. Moving with control, sweep your left leg under you and back to a kneeling position. Take the time here to find a good position, with your left knee pointing toward your left wrist. It's worth saying again that the right arm holding the kettlebell must remain vertical and that the right elbow and wrist must remain locked and straight.

6. Using your left arm and hips, push yourself up into to a lunge/kneeling position. Square yourself off, with your right leg forward and your left leg down. Take your time and adjust your feet if necessary to find 90° angles of the knees, ankles, and right hip (tucking the toes of the back foot). Your right arm should be close to your ear and vertical. Shift your eyes to the horizon. Stand up strongly by pressing through your planted foot and assisting with your back leg.

7. Now all that's left is to reverse the steps. Remember that all rules of muscle engagement and joint positions still apply! Stepping back with your left leg into a lunge, sink your hips straight down until your knee is on the floor. "Windshield wiper" your back foot underneath you and then hinge at the hip, finding the floor with your left hand. Sweep your left leg through, and carefully lower your hips to the floor. Lower your elbow to the floor while keeping your shoulders down, and roll down to your back and slightly toward your left side. Put both hands on the kettlebell, and lower it to your chest. Roll to your right side to place the kettlebell down.

8.   Repeat on your left side.

Note: There are no separate levels shown on the following pages, just the one full sequence.

The following photos are shown using a shoe instead of a Kettlebell. This is the beginner level. Once you have learned the movement thoroughly and can stabilize a Kettlebell overhead you may start to use a light Kettlebell.

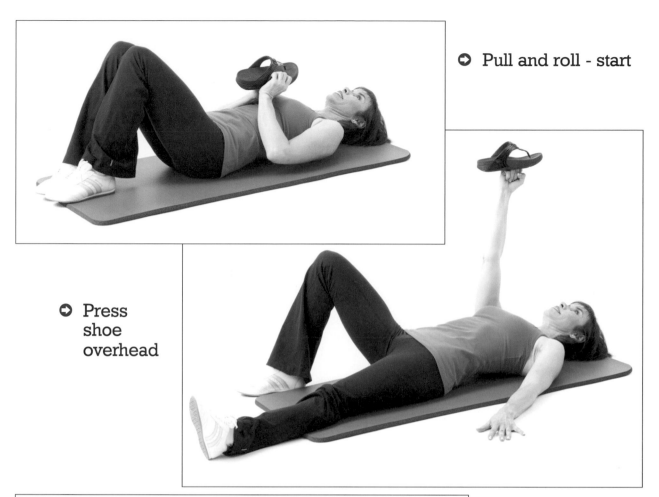

○ Pull and roll - start

○ Press
shoe
overhead

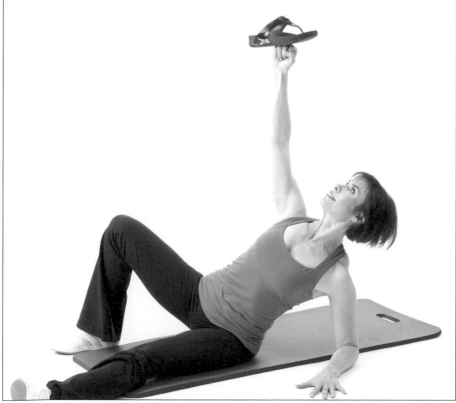

○ To elbow

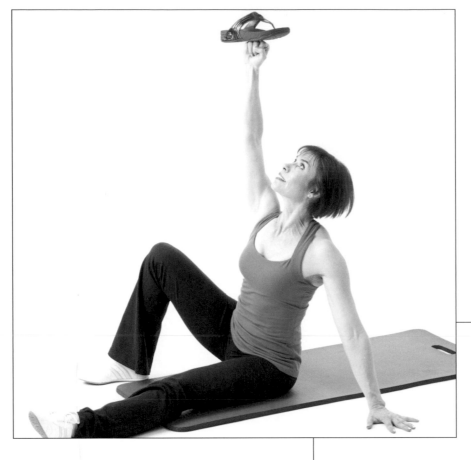

➲ To hand

Note: There are two safe ways to prepare for a get-up on your left side from here. One is to perform a halo motion with the kettlebell, dragging it on the ground behind your head. The other is simply to spin your body 180° and then roll to your left side to face the kettlebell.

➲ Leg sweep

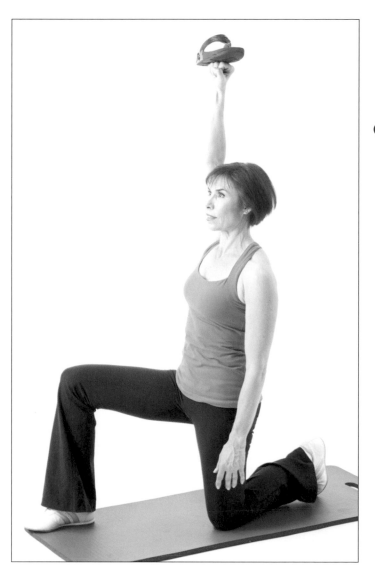

➲ Lunge

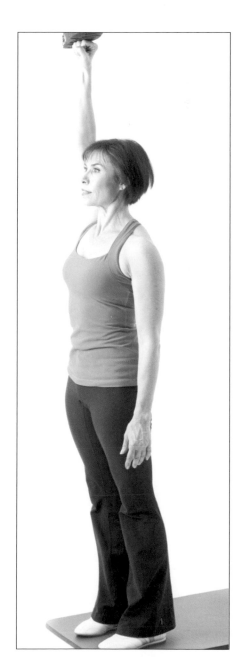

➲ Stand up

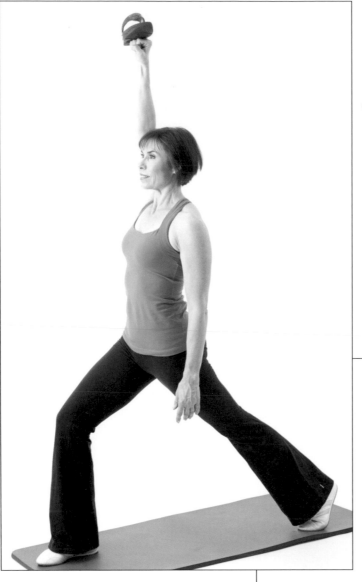

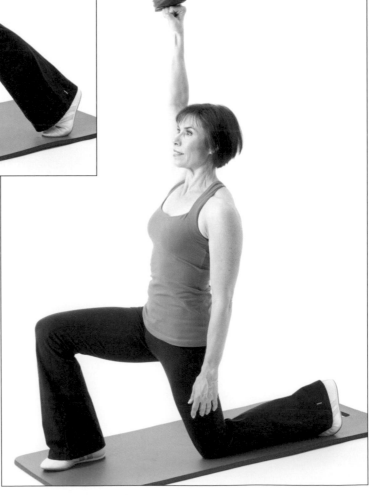

● Step back into lunge

● Lower to knee

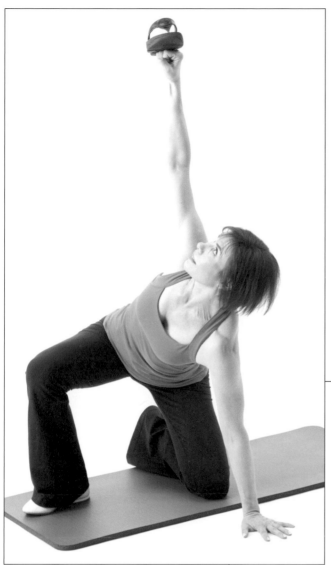

➡ Sweep leg back

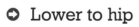 Lower to hip

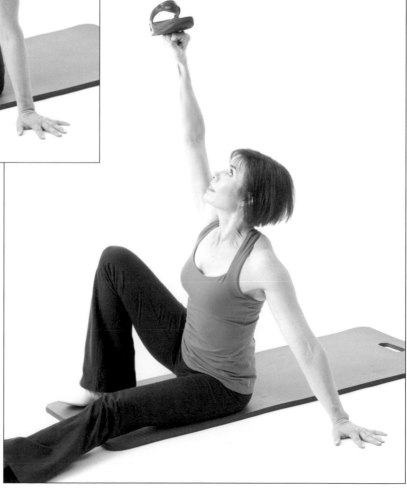

⮕ Lower to elbow

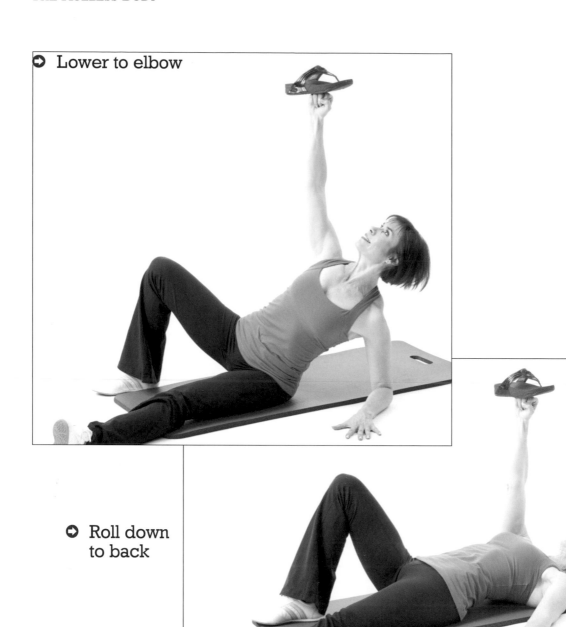

⮕ Roll down
  to back

⮕ Lower shoe
  or KB with
  both hands

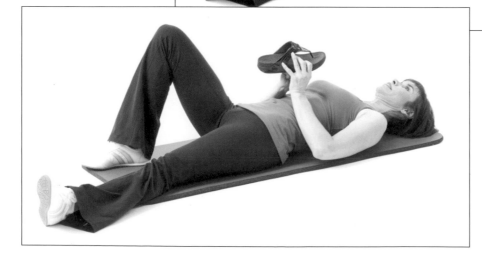

Chapter 9

Balance Drills

Having good balance is the key to preventing falls by the elderly. Maintaining the strength and stability to stand on one leg is one of the most important factors in reducing seniors' falls, and even young and otherwise active people can have difficulty standing on one leg. Performing the following drills is a simple way to train your stabilizing muscles and to develop the strength to maintain balance on one leg.

NO WEIGHT, USING A CHAIR
Key Points:

1. Stand next to a chair, holding on to it lightly with one hand.

2. Shift all of your weight to one leg, and lift your hand away from the chair for 10 to 30 seconds. Repeat on the other side.

3. Be conscious that you are pulling up your kneecaps and thigh muscles.

4. Squeeze your glutes tight, and keep your abs engaged.

5. Lengthen your spine by pressing your head to the ceiling and lifting your sternum.

6. Repeat on both sides, but this time, try to lift one leg off of the ground and hold your balance for 10 to 30 seconds. Hold on to the chair only as needed.

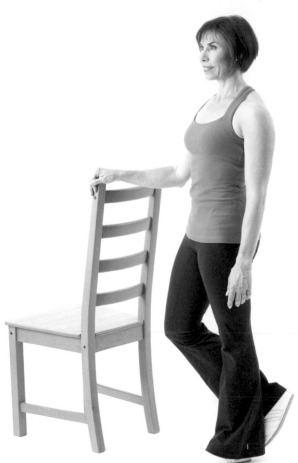

➲ No weight, using
chair (1 - Beg)

➲ No weight, using
chair (2 - Beg)

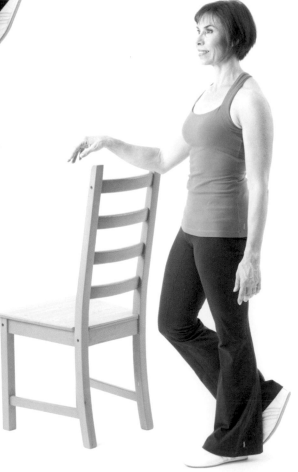

HOLDING THE KETTLEBELL AT THE SIDE

Key Points:

1. You may hold on to a chair in the beginning if necessary.

2. Safely pick up a kettlebell, as if you are getting ready to do a "farmer's walk."

3. Make sure to lift your shoulder up and then down and back, squeezing your lats.

4. Keep your abs engaged, squeeze your glutes tight, pull up your kneecaps, and lengthen your spine.

5. Shift your weight to one leg (and attempt to lift your foot off of the floor, if you can), and take your hand away from the chair for 10 to 30 seconds.

6. Switch legs by doing a perfect suitcase deadlift and switching arms with the kettlebell. Repeat on the other side.

○ **Chair with KB (1 - Adv/Beg)**   ○ **Chair with KB (2 - Adv/Beg)**

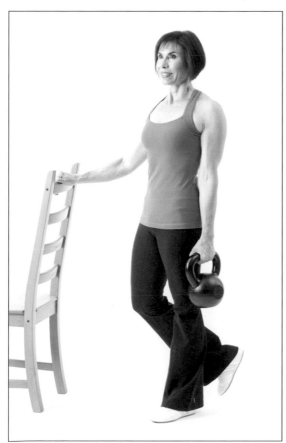
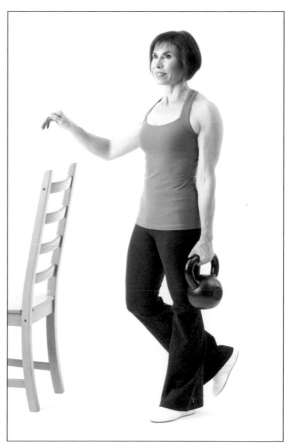

HOLDING THE KETTLEBELL OVERHEAD
Key Points:

1. Clean and press the kettlebell overhead.

2. Squeeze your glutes tight, pull up your kneecaps, and lengthen your spine.

3. Lift your opposite foot off the floor and hold. (You will be holding the kettlebell using the arm on the same side as the leg that you are standing on.) Switch arms and legs.

4. You may also hold the kettlebell in the arm opposite the leg you are standing on.

5. All of the other points apply for performing the military press.

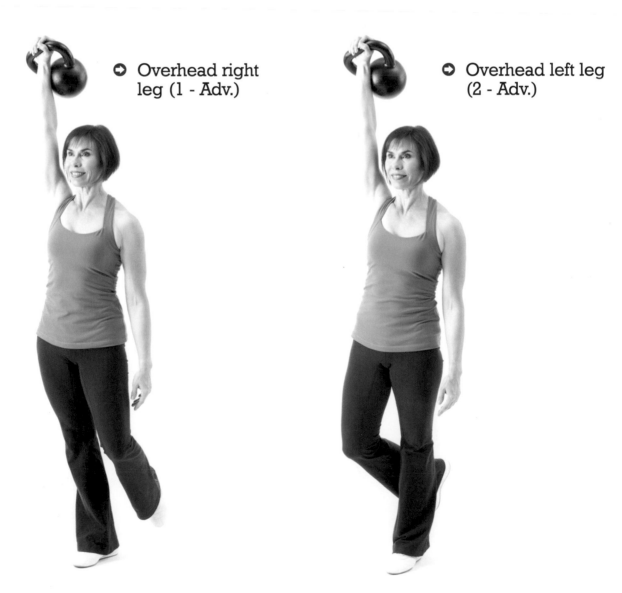

⇨ Overhead right leg (1 - Adv.)

⇨ Overhead left leg (2 - Adv.)

Chapter 10

Cool-Down Stretches

HIP FLEXOR STRETCH
From the Floor
Key Points:

1. Start by kneeling on a soft surface, with one leg forward and your hips squared straight ahead and level.

2. Your legs should be hip distance apart and follow imaginary parallel lines.

3. Place your hands on your hips or the small of your back.

4. Squeeze your glutes and push forward with your pelvis, simultaneously reaching your head to the ceiling and lengthening your spine.

5. Do not allow your forward knee to travel over your toes.

6. Keep your eyes level, or look slightly up.

7. Exhale as you go forward, and inhale as you come back up. Repeat this a few times, moving in and out of the stretch in a gentle rhythm.

8. Repeat on your other leg.

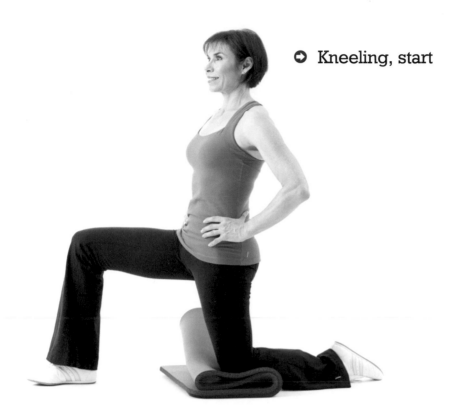

● Kneeling, start

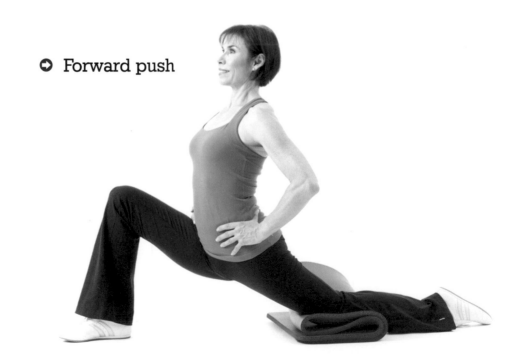

● Forward push

Using a Chair
Key Points:

1. Stand next to a sturdy chair. Hang on to the back for balance.

2. Place your right foot on the seat of the chair.

3. Keep your legs and feet hip distance apart.

4. Push yourself forward, keeping your back leg straight.

5. Do not let your forward knee go over your toes.

6. Lengthen your spine as you go forward.

7. Keep your eyes level, or look slightly up.

8. Exhale as you go forward, and inhale as you come back up. Repeat this a few times, moving in and out of the stretch.

9. Switch legs and repeat.

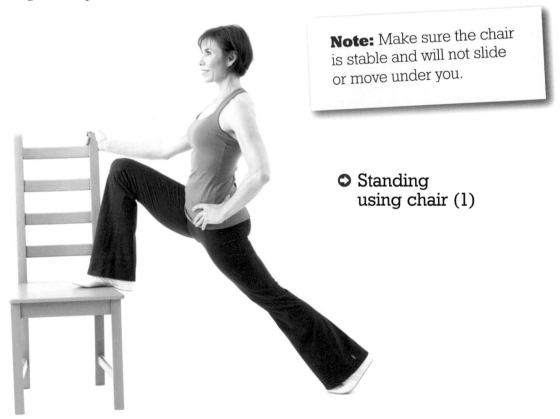

Note: Make sure the chair is stable and will not slide or move under you.

➲ Standing
   using chair (1)

HALF-PIGEON/FIGURE 4
Seated on the Floor
Key Points:

1. Lie on your back.

2. Cross your left ankle over and on to your right knee.

3. Pull your right knee into your chest, grabbing it with both hands.

4. You may grab around your right thigh instead of your knee if necessary.

5. Keep your left knee pushing out to the side, pointing away from you.

6. Rock back and forth to create a rhythmic stretch.

7. Repeat on both sides.

➲ Sitting on floor (1)

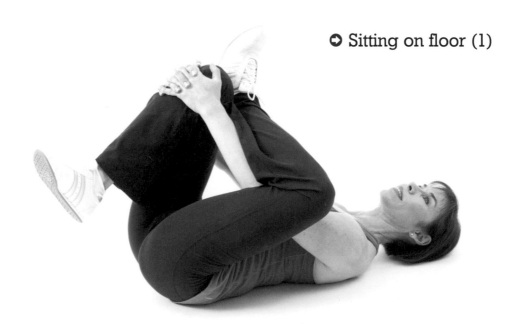

Seated on a chair
Key Points:

1. Sit tall on a chair.

2. Cross your left ankle over and on to your right knee.

3. Drop your left knee down, opening up your hips.

4. Press and release your left leg to increase and decrease the stretch.

5. Make sure you are sitting tall on your "sits bones."

6. Repeat on both sides.

➲ Sitting on chair (1)

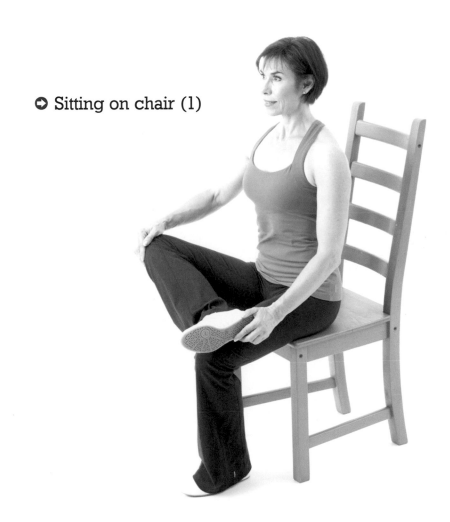

Half Pigeon from the Floor
Key Points:

1. Sit on the floor, and extend your right leg behind you.

2. Tuck your left leg in front and across your body.

3. If possible, have your shin perpendicular to your midline.

4. Keep your left foot flexed.

5. Lean forward over your front (left) leg.

6. Repeat on the other side.

➲ Half Pigeon on floor

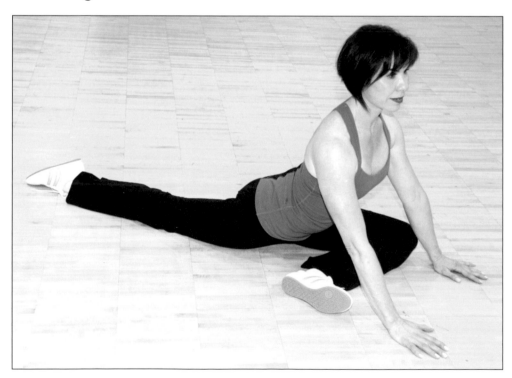

QUAD STRETCH
From the Floor
Key Points:

1. Sit on the floor.

2. Bend your right leg behind you.

3. Push your right hip forward as you keep your right knee back and on the floor.

4. If you are very flexible, lean back and drop onto your elbows.

5. Repeat on the other side.

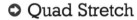

❍ **Quad Stretch**

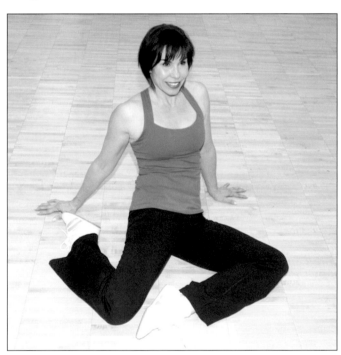

From Standing
Key Points:

1. Hold on to a chair or wall.

2. Standing on your left leg, reach behind you and grab your right ankle, shin, or foot, whichever is most comfortable.

3. Pull your leg up and behind you, keeping your knees close together.

4. Push your hips forward, squeeze your glutes tight, and stand up tall while gently pulling back on the right leg.

5. Try not to lean forward with your upper body. Also try to keep your knees next to each other, so that your bent leg is not too far in front of or behind your standing leg.

6. Repeat on the other side.

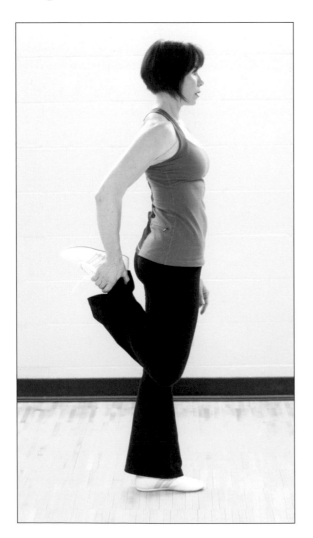

➲ Standing Quad Stretch

HAMSTRING STRETCH
From the Floor with a Band or Strap
Key Points:

1. Sit on the floor.

2. Bend your right leg behind you.

3. Push your right hip forward as you keep your right knee back and on the floor.

4. If you are very flexible, lean back and drop onto your elbows.

5. Repeat on the other side.

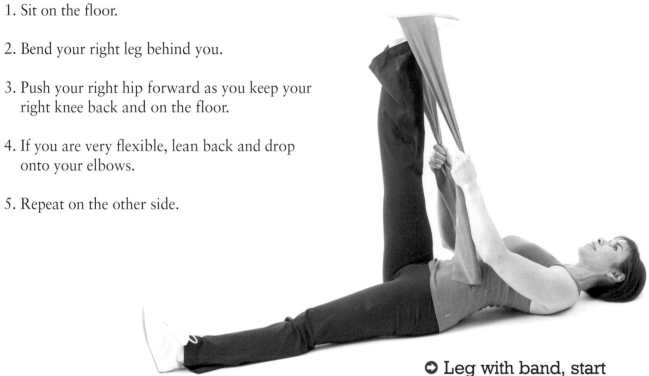

⮕ Leg with band, start

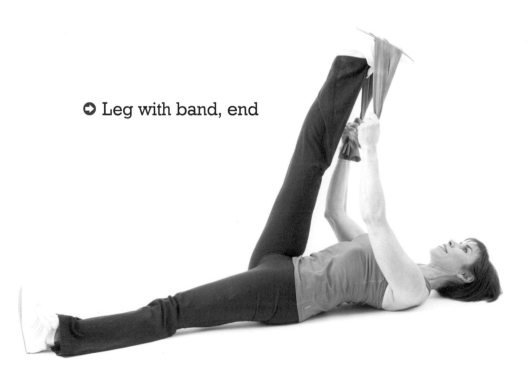

⮕ Leg with band, end

Standing with Leg on Chair
Key Points:

1. Hold on to a chair or wall.

2. Standing on your left leg, reach behind you and grab your right ankle, shin, or foot, whichever is most comfortable.

3. Pull your leg up and behind you, keeping your knees close together.

4. Push your hips forward, squeeze your glutes tight, and stand up tall while gently pulling back on the right leg.

5. Try not to lean forward with your upper body. Also try to keep your knees next to each other, so that your bent leg is not too far in front of or behind your standing leg.

6. Repeat on the other side.

➲ Leg on chair

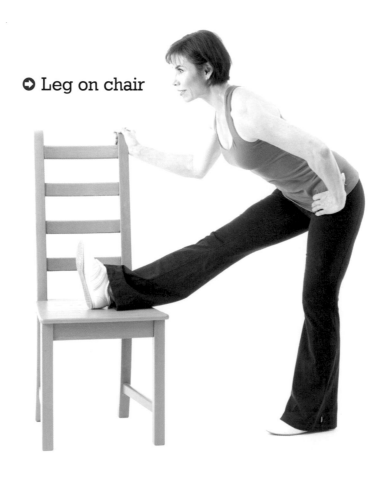

Runner's Stretch
Key Points:

1. Sit on the floor with your right leg straight out in front of you and your left leg tucked in.

2. Keep your right knee straight, and flex your right foot up.

3. Reach both hands out and over the leg, reaching for your right foot, ankle, or shin.

4. Push your left knee to the floor if possible.

5. Repeat on the other side.

○ Runner's Stretch

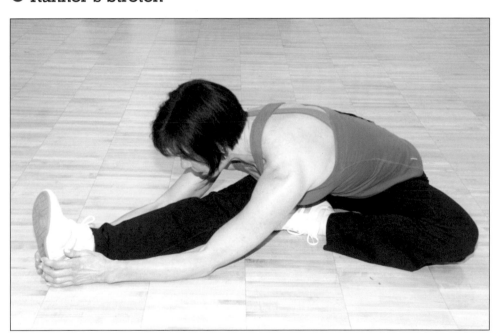

T-SPINE ROTATION
Key Points:

1. Lay on the floor on your right side. Bring both knees toward your chest, and then hold them to the ground with your right hand.

2. With your left hand, reach across your chest to grab hold of your ribcage.

3. Turn your head and look left with your eyes, pulling your chest left and open on the exhale.

4. Breathe and look with the movement. Exhale as you pull your ribcage, looking left, and inhale as you release, allowing your spine (including your neck) to return to neutral.

5. Repeat on both sides.

⊙ T-Spint Rotation on floor

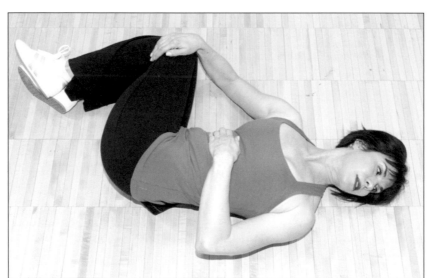

With an Arm Sweep
Key Points:

1. Extend your left arm flat on the floor and 90° to the side (straight off your shoulder).

2. With each inhale, sweep your arm up toward your ear as far as you can, while keeping your hand (palm up), wrist, elbow, and shoulder flat on the floor.

3. Exhale, and return your arm to the starting position.

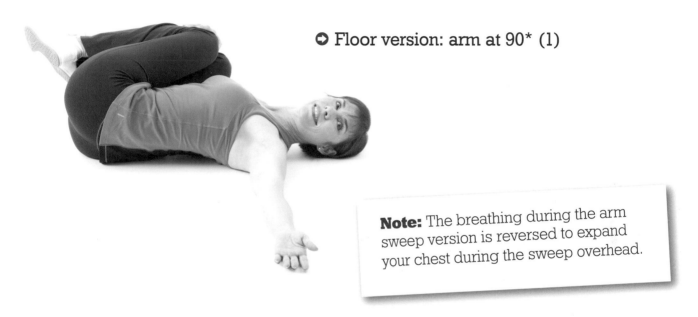

→ Floor version: arm at 90* (1)

Note: The breathing during the arm sweep version is reversed to expand your chest during the sweep overhead.

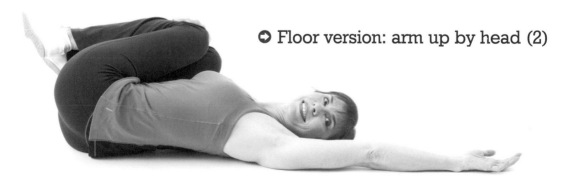

→ Floor version: arm up by head (2)

SEATED PUSH/PULL
Key Points:

1. Sit sideways on a chair that has a back.

2. Sit tall, with your right side facing the chair.

3. Make sure you are sitting on your "sits bones" and keeping your knees together.

4. Grab hold of the back of the chair with both hands.

5. Use your hands to push/pull yourself into more rotation. Get as much rotation as you can without moving your hips or pelvis.

6. Exhale as you rotate, and inhale as you relax.

7. Stay tall. Do not slouch or round your lower back.

8. Repeat on both sides.

○ Seated version: Push/pull

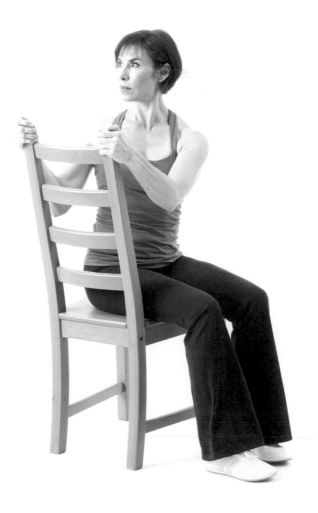

With an Arm Sweep
Key Points:

1.   While rotating, extend your right arm and sweep it up.

2.   Breathe in as your arm goes up, and breathe out as it goes down.

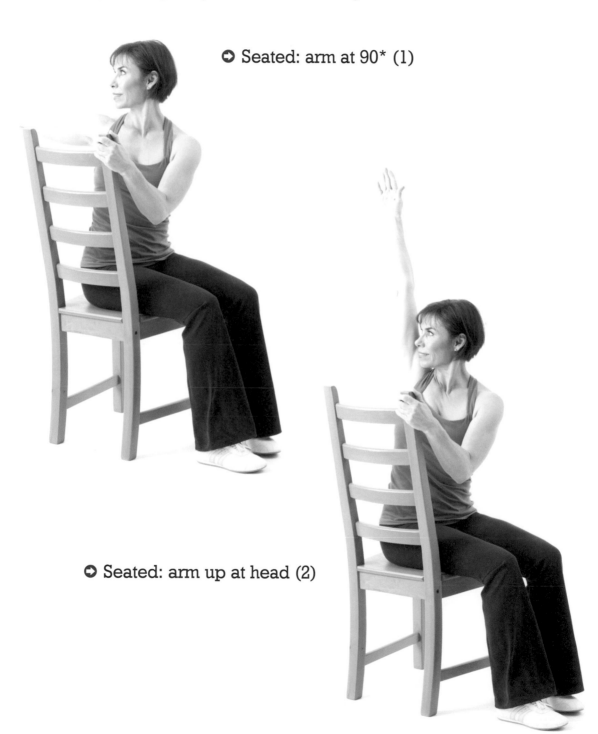

⊃ Seated: arm at 90* (1)

⊃ Seated: arm up at head (2)

Down Dog
Hands on the Floor
Key Points:

1. On a nonskid surface (such as a yoga mat), place your hands on the floor in front of you, shoulder width apart.

2. Place your feet hip width apart.

3. Keep your elbows and knees straight, and push your chest down.

4. Reach your heels to the floor. They do not have to touch the floor, however.

5. Pull up your kneecaps.

6. Try to press your hips up toward the ceiling and to maintain a straight back. You may slightly bend your knees if necessary.

7. Keep your head in line with your back.

○ Down Dog on floor

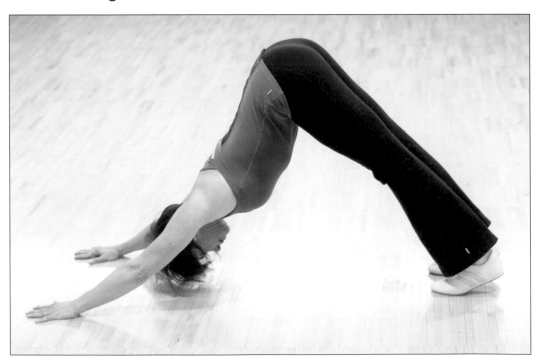

Using a Chair

Key Points:

1. Grab on to a high-backed, sturdy chair with both hands.
2. Place your feet hip distance apart, and push your hips back, keeping your arms straight.
3. Let your knees bend as much as needed.
4. Keep your head in line with your back.

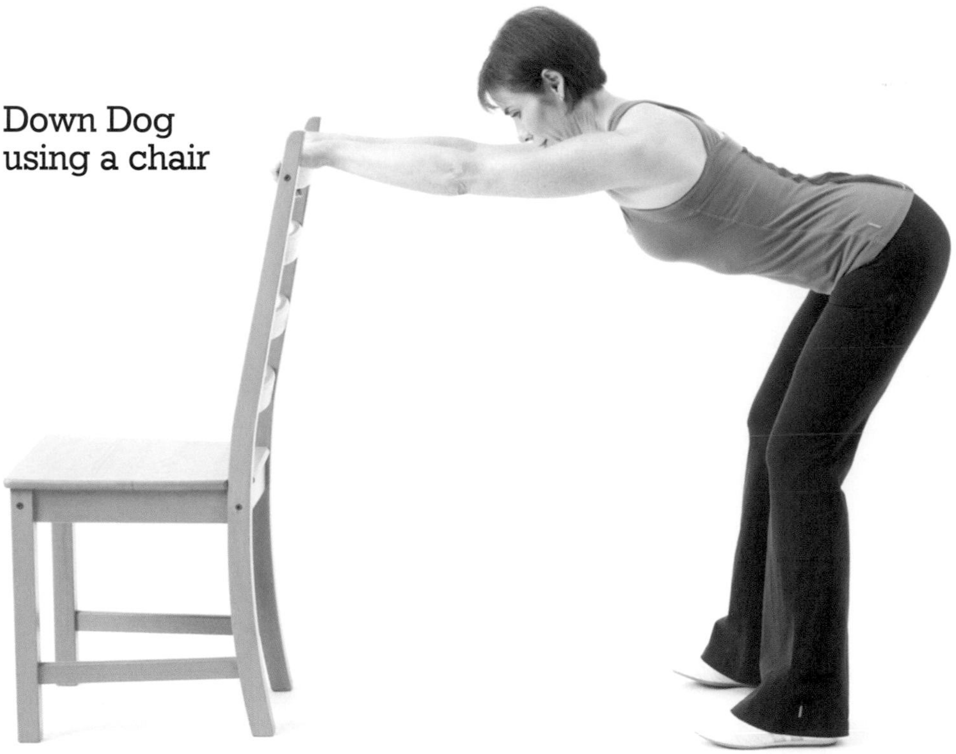

➲ Down Dog using a chair

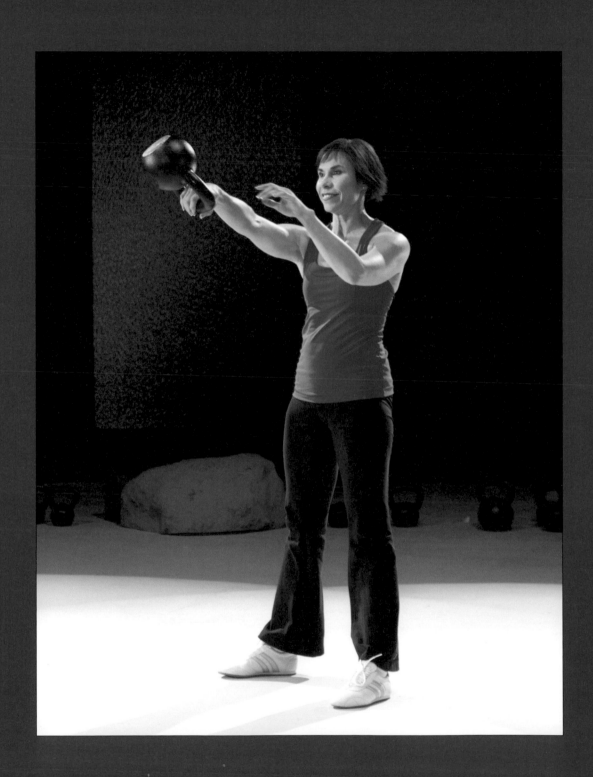

Chapter 11

Advanced Kettlebell Exercises

This section of exercises is for those who have been training with kettlebells for some time and so have learned proper and safe technique and developed adequate strength to perform the drills safely. I highly recommend that you get your form checked by a certified RKC instructor before attempting these advanced drills on your own.

CLEAN

Single Kettlebell Clean

Key Points:

1. Begin the clean the same as the swing, but bend your arm and pull it into your body at the top. Do not shrug your shoulder to accomplish this.

2. At the top, the kettlebell, your arm, and your body become one. They must connect at the same time. Your shoulders should be pressed down, your wrist straight, and your arm in contact with your ribcage. The kettlebell should be nested between your upper and lower arm.

3. To reclean the kettlebell, think of "spilling" the kettlebell forward by turning your wrist slightly and then pulling your hips back, as in the swing.

4. The lower part of the movement is exactly the same as the swing. Hike the kettlebell high up between your legs and toward your tailbone. As you reach, hinge your hips back. It helps to rotate your forearm inward during the backswing. (For clarification on this, read points 2 and 3 of the following section on the double swing.)

5. Your hips should do all of the work; your arms only guide and rack the kettlebell. Your arms must remain loose while the kettlebell is in motion.

6. Keep the arc of the kettlebell close to your body throughout the movement, as though there is an imaginary wall in front of you that you may not hit.

7. Make sure you DO NOT do any of the following: bang your forearms, curl the kettlebell up, allow your wrist to bend at the top, scoop your hips, or use your arms to lift the kettlebell in any way.

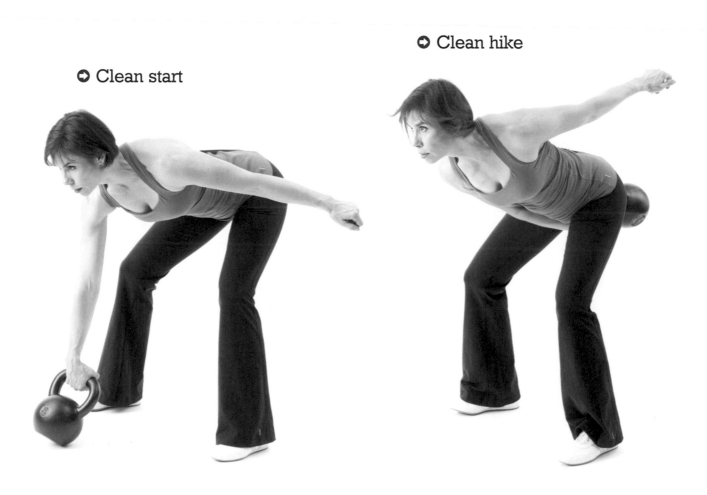

➲ Clean start

➲ Clean hike

6. Keep the arc of the kettlebell close to your body throughout the movement, as though there is an imaginary wall in front of you that you may not hit.

7. Make sure you DO NOT do any of the following: bang your forearms, curl the kettlebell up, allow your wrist to bend at the top, scoop your hips, or use your arms to lift the kettlebell in any way.

⊃ Clean pull

⊃ Clean end

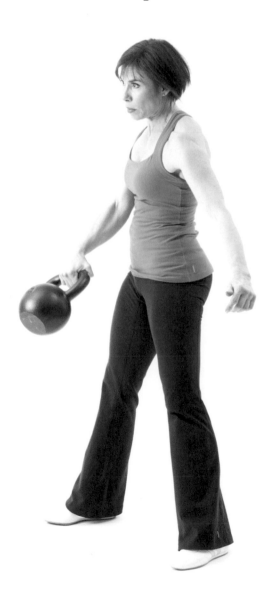
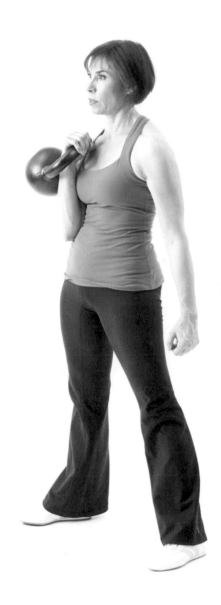

DOUBLE SWING

Key Points:

1. Take a slightly wider stance than for the single clean.

2. Rotate the handles of the kettlebells so that when you look down at them on the ground, they form a V shape.

3. Rotate the backs of your hands together as you pull the kettlebells between your legs.

4. Always perform a strong hike pass between your legs.

5. Keep your elbows straight.

6. Keep your weight back on your heels throughout the swing. Resist the tendency to be pulled forward that comes with using double kettlebells.

7. Keep your chest up, and look forward at the bottom.

● DB Swing start

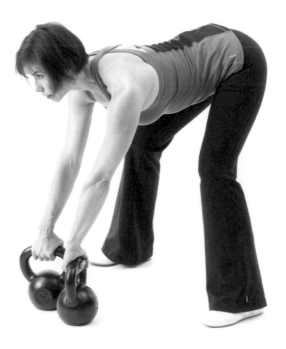

8. Pinch your shoulder blades together and keep your shoulders tightly down throughout.

9. Do not swing higher than chest height.

10. Do not fail to hinge at the hips during the backswing. A common mistake is to keep your body too vertical, which eliminates the benefits of the hike pass.

11. All other points about the single clean apply to performing the double swing.

DB Swing hike

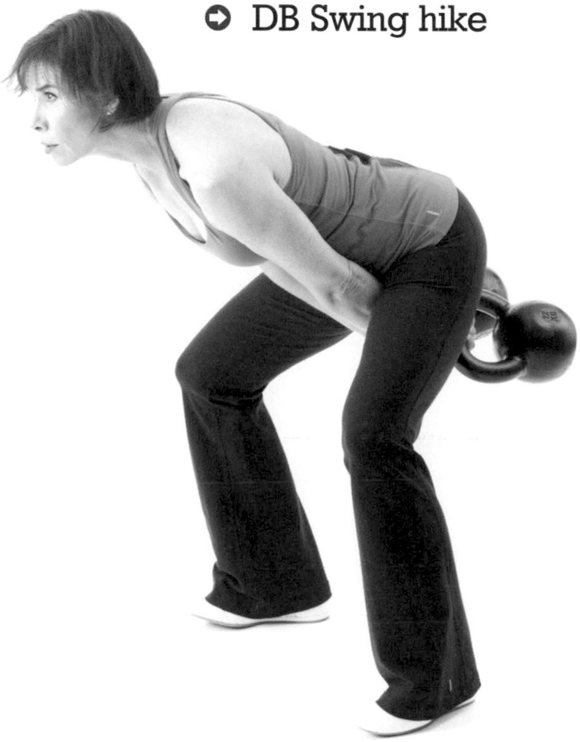

DB Swing top

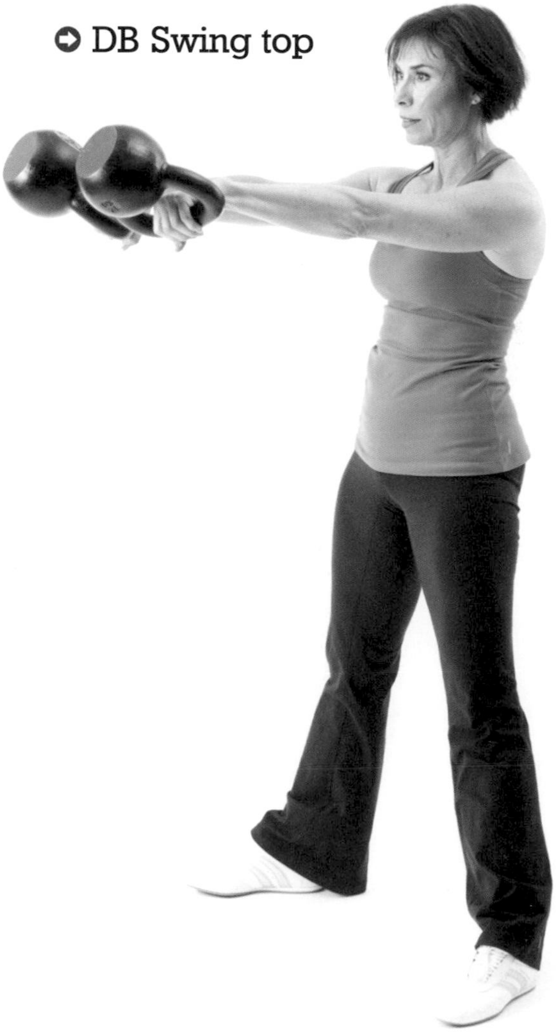

DOUBLE CLEAN
Key Points:

1. Instead of keeping your elbows straight, bend them to pull the kettlebell into your chest. Do not shrug your shoulders to accomplish this.

2. Imagine that you are cleaning to your waist, not to your chest.

3. Actively squeeze your arms against your body at the top.

◐ DB Clean start

◐ DB Clean hike

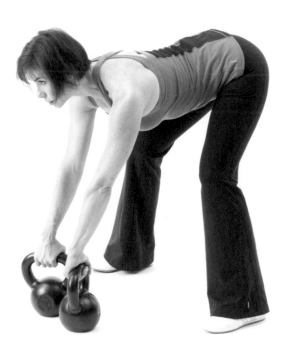

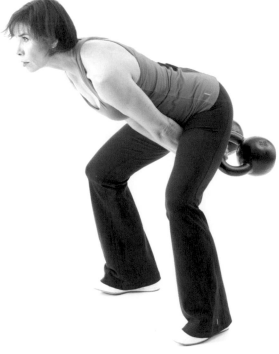

4. Open your fingers at the top to prevent hitting your fingers between the handles.

5. Do not cast the kettlebells forward. Keep your arms relaxed and the kettlebells close, and then throw them back into the hike position.

6. All other points about the single clean and double swing apply to performing the double clean.

⊙ **DB Clean pull**   ⊙ **DB Clean end**

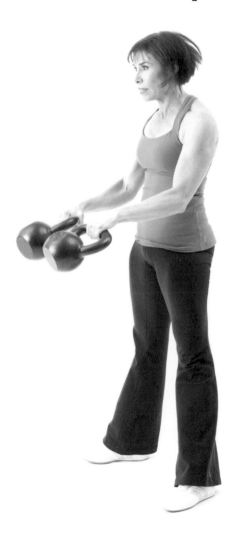
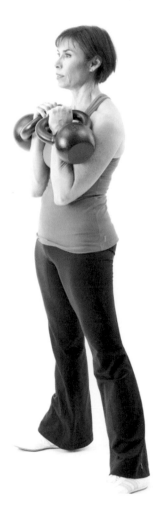

DOUBLE PRESS
Key Points:

1. Take a slightly wider stance the same as in double swings.

2. Rotate the handles of the kettlebells so that when you look down at them on the ground, they form a V shape.

3. Rotate the backs of your hands together as you pull the kettlebells between your legs.

4. Instead of keeping your elbows straight, bend them to pull the kettlebell into your chest. Do not shrug your shoulders to accomplish this.

5. Start to press with your fists at collarbone level, your kneecaps pulled up, your glutes squeezed tight, and your abs engaged.

➲ From clean position, start

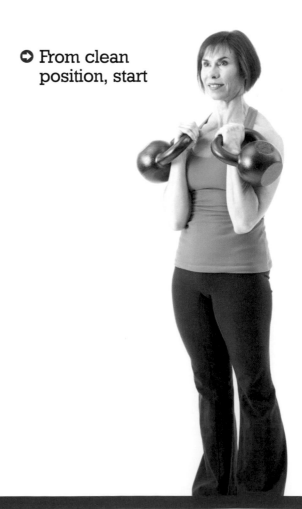

6. Keep your forearms vertical throughout the movement.

7. Keep your shoulders down. Do not let them shrug up, toward your ears.

8. Lock out your elbow to finish at the top. Your arms should be near your ears and your shoulders packed.

9. Power breathe. DO NOT exhale completely during the press. You may inhale slightly at the top and then hiss out more air on the descent.

10. When lowering the kettlebells, keep your body tight and grounded. You may slowly pull the kettlebells toward you, as if you are doing a chin-up (advanced), or simply control its descent.

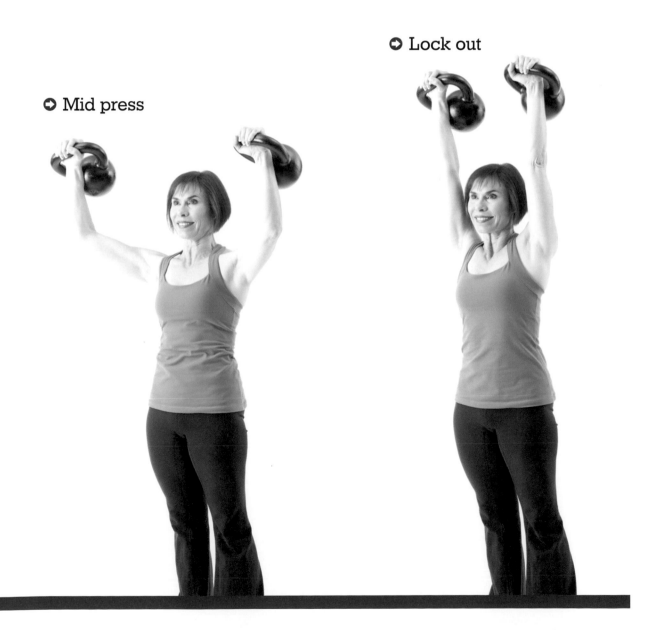

○ Lock out

○ Mid press

FRONT SQUAT
Key Points:

1. Double clean your kettlebells into the rack position without banging your wrists or letting the kettlebells push you backward.

2. You may adjust your feet to achieve your optimal squat position, but do not lose tension.

3. Pull your shoulders down, and keep your arms against your ribcage.

4. Men may lace their fingers together before squatting.

5. Women must not press the kettlebells against their breasts. They may have to hold the kettlebells more out to the sides, which will not allow as much of the abdominal pressure that men get.

6. Inhale sharply and deeply through your nose, and pull yourself down with your hip flexors. Keep as tight as possible, especially your abdominals and obliques.

7. At the bottom, pause briefly. While keeping tight, grunt to start the ascent, and then finish with crisp hips.

8. Keep your spine tall throughout the exercise, and never squat deeper than the level at which you can maintain a straight back.

9. All other points about the goblet squat apply to performing the front squat. The difference is in the double kettlebell rack position.

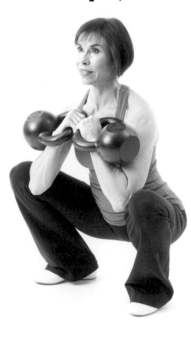

➲ Front Squat, bottom

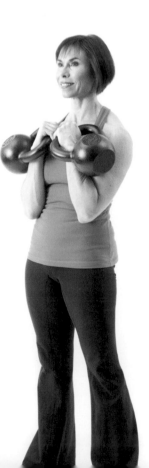

➲ Front Squat, start

GOBLET SQUAT WITH A CURL

Key Points:

1. Start from the bottom of the goblet squat, your elbows pressing against the insides of your knees.

2. Keeping your body and elbows in place, lower the kettlebell until your arms lock out.

3. Continue to think of lengthening your spine and reaching with the crown of your head, allowing yourself to sink deeper. Your lower back should not round, and your hips should not scoop under.

4. Curl the kettlebell back into the goblet squat position.

5. Repeat.

6. All other points about the front squat apply to performing this squat.

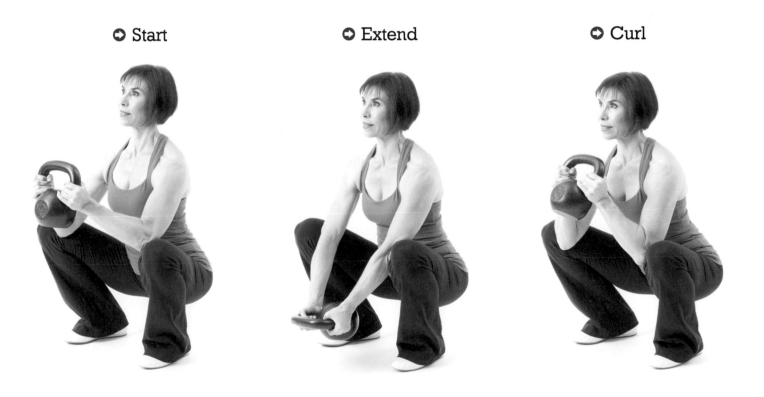

➲ Start   ➲ Extend   ➲ Curl

GOBLET SQUAT WITH A FRONT RAISE

Key Points:

1. Start from the bottom of the goblet squat position, your elbows pressing against the insides of your knees.

2. Keeping your body and elbows in place, lower the kettlebell until your arms lock out.

3. With your arms straight, slowly raise the kettlebell overhead. Allow your hips to sink.

4. Keep your chest lifted and your chin level.

5. When your arms cannot go any further, maintain your upper body in this position and squat up.

6. Return the kettlebell to the goblet squat position, and then squat back down to set up for another repetition.

7. ll other points about the front squat apply to performing this squat.

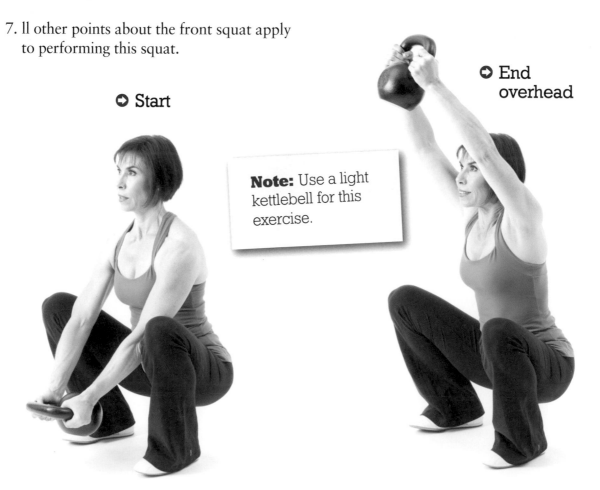

➲ Start

Note: Use a light kettlebell for this exercise.

➲ End overhead

SNATCH
Key Points:

1. The snatch begins the same as the swing and then travels close to the body, as in the clean, before locking out overhead. (The snatch ends in the same overhead position as though you have pressed a kettlebell overhead.)

2. Strongly hike the kettlebell back, rotating your forearm in slightly as it travels behind you.

3. Imagine performing a powerful swing, but then keep the kettlebell close to your body and punch your arm overhead. Your shoulder should not shrug to accomplish this, and your arm should only guide the kettlebell into the lockout, not press it up.

Note: This is an extremely advanced and tricky exercise to learn on your own. I highly recommend that you see a certified RKC instructor to help learn this technique. I also recommend getting a copy of Pavel's *Enter the Kettlebell!* Book or DVD for further instruction.

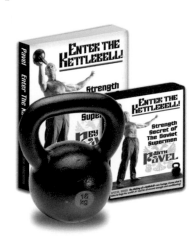

⊙ Start

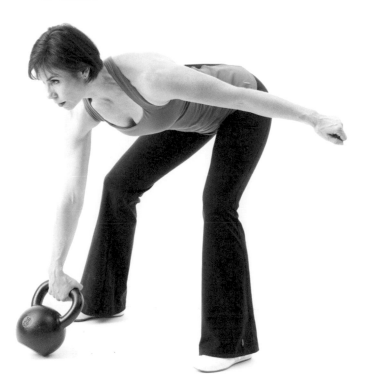

⊙ Hike

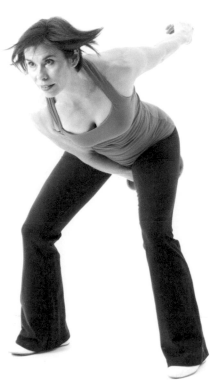

4. In flight, the kettlebell will rotate over your wrist as you spear your hand directly up (as though punching the ceiling). The kettlebell should land softly, without banging your forearm or jarring your shoulder.

5. Your arm must lock out by your head or ear. Your elbow should be locked and your wrist straight, with your shoulder pulled down.

6. Your body, arm, and feet must be motionless for a second at the top, and your legs must be straight.

7. Lower the kettlebell in one smooth motion. Keep it as close to your body as possible, without touching your chest or shoulder.

8. The kettlebell should end as far back between your legs and close to your body as possible, loading your hips as much as possible for the next rep.

9. Use biomechanical breathing to encourage explosive power of your hips.

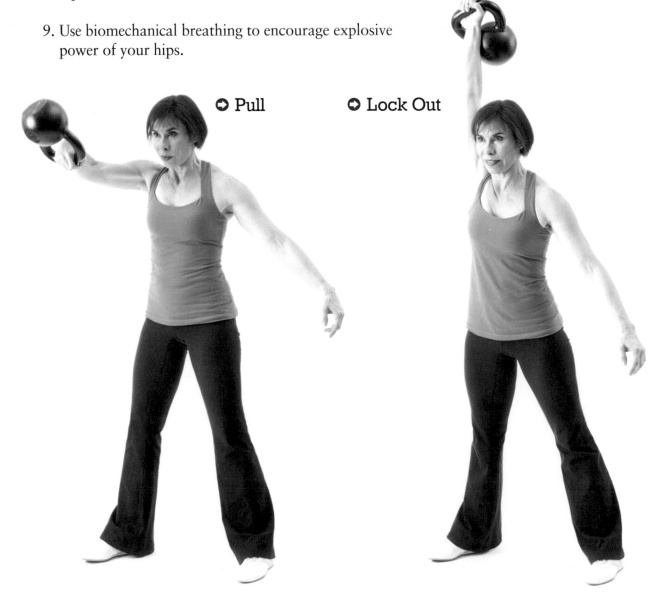

⮕ Pull ⮕ Lock Out

Part III

Workouts

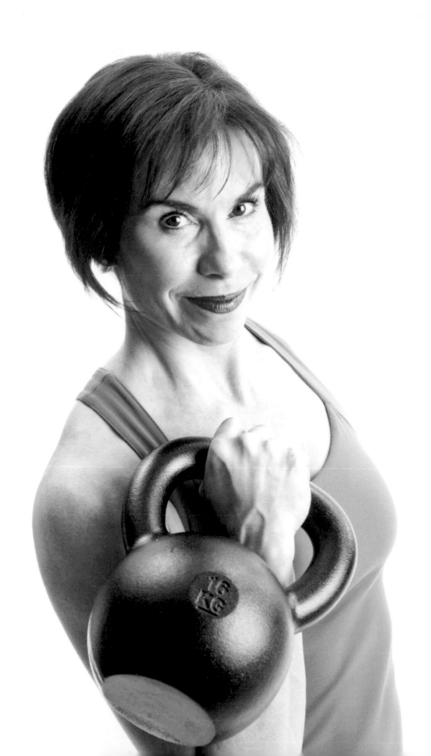

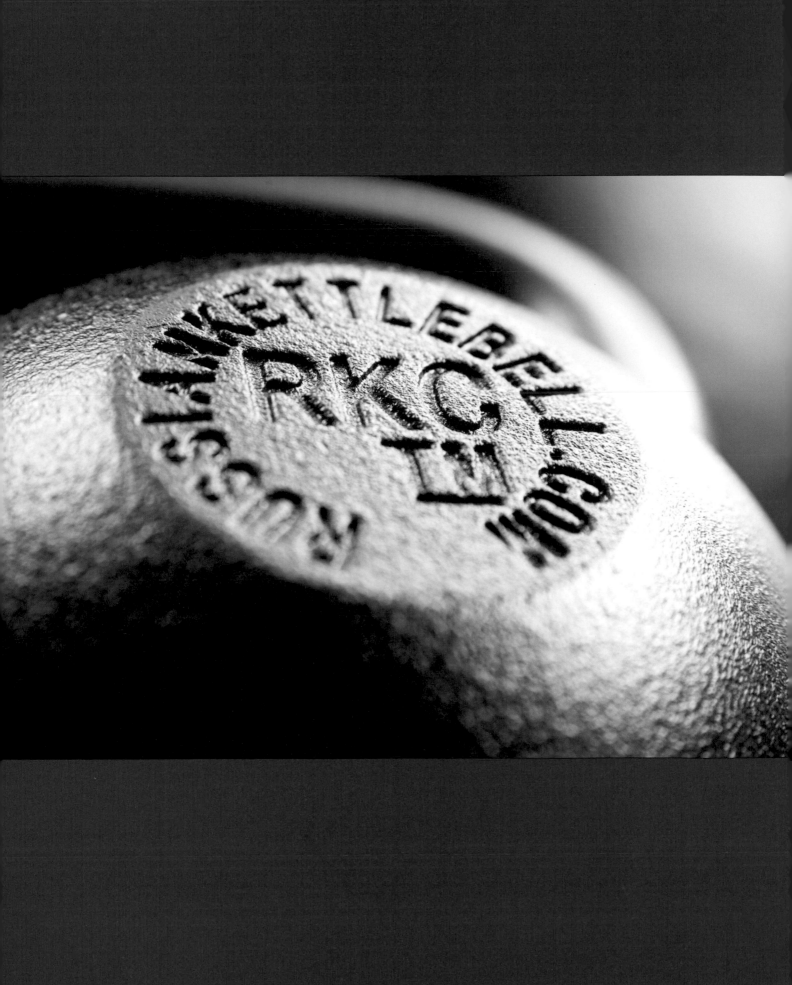

Chapter 12

Planning Your Workouts

First and foremost, you should build up slowly. For the first couple of weeks, focus on perfecting the prep drills and spend some time working on your mobility and flexibility.

Next, focus on learning each exercise in the book. As you may notice, the exercises are taught in a way that builds you up safely, starting with all the variations of the deadlift and then moving on to the plank, the swing, and so on. Once you have learned one exercise, you will be ready to move on to the next exercise in the book. Plan to spend a week focusing on each drill before moving on to the next one.

Make sure you start each practice with the warm-up. Then move on to the exercise you are working on that day, and finish with the cool-down. For example, your first few workouts might look like this:

Warm-up for approximately 10 minutes
Practice deadlifts for 15–20 minutes
Finish with cool-down stretches for 5–10 minutes

During the instructional phase, your workouts should end up being around 30 minutes long.

By the time you have gone through all of the drills a few times, you will have slowly built up your strength and stamina. Doing so will allow you to follow the workouts both safely and more easily.

Make sure you are completely comfortable with your particular level of each exercise before attempting to follow either workout. Once you have learned all the exercises and feel confident about doing them, you will be ready to begin working out. Feel free to design your own workout once you feel comfortable with all the drills.

You will start with the Six-Week Ramp-Up in Chapter 13. Once you have completed this initial program, then move on to the Sample Six-Week Workout, found later in that chapter.

Six-Week Ramp-Up & Sample Six-Week Program

You are now ready to begin doing a workout. Remember that you should spend as much time as necessary to learn each drill thoroughly before attempting to follow a workout. It doesn't matter if you start with the strength or cardio workout. Doing either one will give you a balanced, full-body workout.

Make sure you have everything you need at hand before you start to work out, including the following:

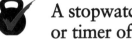 A stopwatch, Gymboss, or timer of some sort

 A chair

 A platform if necessary

 Plenty of water

If you are completely new to exercising, start slowly. Maybe do only half of the workout or use half of the allotted time for all of the sets and rounds.

Over time, increase the level you are following as your skill increases. And here are other ideas for increasing the challenge of your workout:

- Increase the number of sets performed during specific rounds.
- Increase the weight used for certain exercises.
- Increase the length of time spent working during sets.
- Decrease the time spent resting between sets.

It's a good idea to change only one of these parameters at a time. For example, something as simple as adding an extra set to one or two rounds or reducing your rest breaks by 5 to 15 seconds during specific rounds will make the workout much more challenging, so don't change too many things at once! As always, build up slowly. And don't be afraid to reduce the challenge of your workout occasionally when you need to.

SIX-WEEK RAMP-UP:
Prepatory and Instructional Phase

Here is a sample Six-Week Prep and Instruction workout, including a warm-up and cool-down:

Week 1

Day 1:	Prep Drills and Balance
Day 2:	Prep Drills and Balance
Day 3:	Deadlift (regular deadlift only)
Day 4:	Plank
Day 5:	Prep Drills and Balance
Day 6:	Deadlift (regular deadlift only)
Day 7:	REST

Week 2

Day 1:	Prep Drills and Balance
Day 2:	Deadlift (regular deadlift only)
Day 3:	Get-Up
Day 4:	Deadlift (add suitcase deadlift)
Day 5:	Plank and Kettlebell Carry
Day 6:	Get-Up
Day 7:	REST

Week 3

Day 1:	Deadlift (regular and suitcase deadlift)
Day 2:	Deadlift (add single leg deadlift)
Day 3:	Plank and Russian Twist
Day 4:	Deadlift and Kettlebell Carry
Day 5:	Get-Up and Balance
Day 6:	Swing
Day 7:	REST

Week 4

Day 1:	Deadlift and Kettlebell Carry
Day 2:	Press
Day 3:	Deadlift and Kettlebell Carry
Day 4:	Swing
Day 5:	Squat and Russian Twist
Day 6:	Swing and Plank
Day 7:	REST

Week 5

Day 1:	Press and Squat
Day 2:	Swing and Plank
Day 3:	Deadlift and Kettlebell Carry
Day 4:	Squat and Russian Twist
Day 5:	Swing and Balance
Day 6:	Press and Squat
Day 7:	REST

Week 6

Day 1:	Swing and Plank
Day 2:	Get-Up
Day 3:	Deadlift and Kettlebell Carry
Day 4:	Press
Day 5:	Swing and Russian Twist
Day 6	Press and Squat
Day 7:	REST

SAMPLE SIX-WEEK PROGRAM:
Overall Strength and Conditioning

The Strength Workout and the Cardio Workout are described in Chapters 15 and 16, respectively.

Week 1

Day 1:   Strength Workout
Day 2:   Warm-Up and Cool-Down only (skip workout)
Day 3:   Cardio Workout
Day 4:   REST
Day 5:   Strength Workout
Day 6:   Get-Up
Day 7:   REST

Week 2

Day 1:   Strength Workout
Day 2:   Warm-Up and Cool-Down only (skip workout)
Day 3:   Cardio Workout
Day 4:   Balance
Day 5:   Strength Workout
Day 6:   Warm-Up and Cool-Down only
Day 7:   REST

Week 3

Day 1:   Cardio Workout
Day 2:   Warm-Up and Cool-Down only (skip workout)
Day 3:   Strength Workout
Day 4:   Get-Up and Balance
Day 5:   Cardio Workout
Day 6:   Warm-Up and Cool-Down only
Day 7:   REST

Week 4

Day 1:   Strength Workout
Day 2:   Warm-Up and Cool-Down only (skip workout)
Day 3:   Cardio Workout
Day 4:   Active Rest (brisk walk, etc.) or Warm-Up and Cool-Down
Day 5:   Strength Workout
Day 6:   Balance
Day 7:   REST

Week 5

Day 1:   Strength Workout
Day 2:   Warm-Up and Cool-Down only (skip workout)
Day 3:   Cardio Workout
Day 4:   Get-Up and Balance
Day 5:   Strength Workout
Day 6:   Warm-Up and Cool-Down only
Day 7:   REST

Week 6

Day 1:   Cardio Workout
Day 2:   Warm-Up and Cool-Down only (skip workout)
Day 3:   Strength Workout
Day 4:   Get-Up and Balance
Day 5:   Cardio Workout
Day 6:   Warm-Up and Cool-Down only
Day 7:   REST

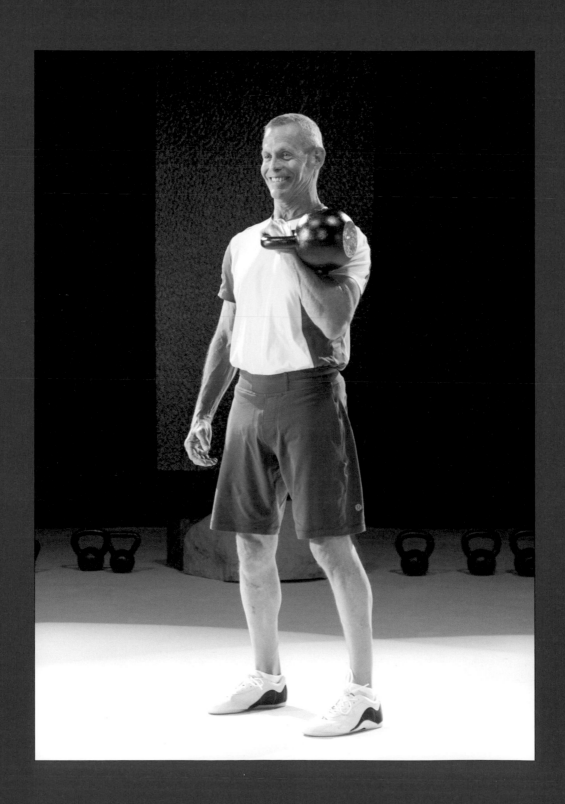

Chapter 14

Strength Workout

pproximate time needed to complete entire workout = 30 minutes

ROUND 1

Do 3 sets, 30 seconds per exercise
No rest

1 set =   Deadlifts 30 seconds
+ Planks 30 seconds

Level	Beginer	Advanced Beginner	Intermediate	Advanced
Deadlifts	Hip hinge, no KB	With platform and KB	From floor with KB	With double KBs
Planks	Wall elbows	Elbows and knees	Elbows and toes	Hands and toes

ROUND 2

Do 2 sets, 30 seconds per exercise
No rest (may rest 10 seconds before kettlebell carries)

1 set =   Right-side suitcase deadlifts 30 seconds
               + Rest 10 seconds
               + Right-side "farmer's walks" 30 seconds
               + Left-side suitcase deadlifts 30 seconds
               + Rest 10 seconds

Note: If using double kettle-bells, try using two different-sized kettlebells from time to time, switching the kettlebells between sets.

Level	Beginer	Advanced Beginner	Intermediate	Advanced
Suitcase Deadlifts	With high platform and KB	With low platform and KB	From floor with KB	With double KBs
Farmer's Walks	Same arm	Same arm	Same arm	Both arms

ROUND 3

Do 2 sets, 30 seconds per side
1:1 work-to-rest ratio

1 set =   Right-side presses 30 seconds
               + Rest 30 seconds
               + Left-side presses 30 seconds
               + Rest 30 seconds

Level	Beginer	Advanced Beginner	Intermediate	Advanced
Presses	Seated assisted	Standing	Kneeling	With one leg on platform

ROUND 4

Do 2 sets, 30 seconds per side
1:1 work-to-rest ratio

Note: Add a hip thrust at the top of each rep.

1 set =   Squats 30 seconds
+ Rest 30 seconds

Level	Beginer	Advanced Beginner	Intermediate	Advanced
Squats	Box squat holding chair	Box squat holding KB	Goblet squat	Double front squat

ROUND 5

Do 2 sets, 30 seconds per side
No rest (may rest 10 seconds before kettlebell carries)

Note: If you are using two kettlebells overhead for your carry, you may lower them into the clean position as needed.

1 set =   Right-side single-leg deadlifts 30 seconds
+ 10 seconds rest
+ Right-side carries 30 seconds
+ Left-side single-leg deadlifts 30 seconds
+ 10 seconds rest
+ Left-side carries 30 seconds

Level	Beginer	Advanced Beginner	Intermediate	Advanced
Single-Leg Deadlifts	Hold chair, no KB	One arm on chair, hold KB with other arm	1 KB	2 KBs
Carries	"Farmer's walk," 1 KB	Hold in clean	1 KB overhead	2 KBs overhead

ROUND 6

Do 2 sets, 30 seconds of work
1:1 work-to-rest ratio

1 set =   Russian twists 30 seconds
+ Rest 30 seconds

Level	Beginer	Advanced Beginner	Intermediate	Advanced
Russian Twists	Seated, no KB	Seated with KB	Standing with KB	Sitting on floor with KB

Chapter 15

Cardio Workout

pproximate time needed to complete entire workout = 30 minutes

ROUND 1

Do 3 sets, 30 seconds of work
1:1 work-to-rest ratio

1 set = Deadlifts 30 seconds
+ Rest 30 seconds

Level	Beginer	Advanced Beginner	Intermediate	Advanced
Deadlifts	Hip hinge, no KB	With platform using KB	From floor with KB	From floor with heavy KB

ROUND 2

Swing for the following durations: 15 seconds, 20 seconds,
30 seconds, 30 seconds,
20 seconds, 15 seconds

1:1 work-to-rest ratio

1 set = One interval of swings followed by
one interval of rest.

Note: Each pair of work
and rest = 1 set.

Level	Beginer	Advanced Beginner	Intermediate	Advanced
Swings	Two-handed	Alternating	One-armed, switch arms each set	With 2 KBs

ROUND 3

Do 1 set, 30 seconds of work
No rest

1 set = Right-side carries 30 seconds
+ Left-side carries 30 seconds

Note: : If you are using two
kettlebells overhead for your
carry, you may lower them into
the clean position as needed.

Level	Beginer	Advanced Beginner	Intermediate	Advanced
Carries	"Farmer's walk" with 1 KB	Hold in clean with 1 KB	1 KB overhead	2 KBs overhead

ROUND 4

Swing for the following durations: 15 seconds, 20 seconds, 30 seconds, 30 seconds, 20 seconds, 15 seconds

1:1 work-to-rest ratio

1 set =   One interval of swings followed by one interval of rest.

Note: Each pair of work and rest = 1 set.

Level	Beginer	Advanced Beginner	Intermediate	Advanced
Swings	Two-handed	Alternating	One-armed, switch arms each set	With 2 KBs

ROUND 5

Do 2 sets, 30 seconds of work
1:1 work-to-rest ratio

1 set =   Squats 30 seconds
+ Rest 30 seconds

Note: Add a hip thrust at the top of each rep.

Level	Beginer	Advanced Beginner	Intermediate	Advanced
Squats	Box squat holding chair	Box squat holding KB	Goblet squat	Double front squat

ROUND 6

Swing for the following durations: 15 seconds, 20 seconds,
30 seconds, 30 seconds,
20 seconds, 15 seconds

1:1 work-to-rest ratio

1 set =   One interval of swings followed by
one interval of rest.

Note: Each pair of work
and rest = 1 set.

Level	Beginer	Advanced Beginner	Intermediate	Advanced
Swings	Two-handed	Alternating	One-armed, switch arms each set	With 2 KBs

ROUND 7

Do 2 sets, 30 seconds of work
1:1 work-to-rest ratio

1 set =   Perform exercise 30 seconds
+ Rest 30 seconds

Level	Beginer	Advanced Beginner	Intermediate	Advanced
Russian Twists	Seated, no KB	Seated with KB	Standing with KB	Sitting on floor with KB

ROUND 8

Do 2 sets, 30 seconds of work
1:1 work-to-rest ratio

1 set =   Squats 30 seconds
+ Rest 30 seconds

Level	Beginer	Advanced Beginner	Intermediate	Advanced
Squats	Box squat holding chair	Box squat holding KB	Goblet squat	Double front squat

Resources

This section provides resources that will help you further your kettlebell quest:

- If you are in need of kettlebells, books, DVDs, or other training resources, the Dragon Door website is the place to go: www.dragondoor.com. This site also has an incredible library full of articles, videos, news updates, online discussion forums, and much more.

- All certified Russian Kettlebell Challenge (RKC) instructors are listed on Dragon Door's website. You should consult one to have your form checked out before attempting the advanced drills on your own. To find an instructor in your area, go to **www.dragondoor.com/rkc/,** and then type in your zip code.

- On the same website, you will find a list of Certified Kettlebell–Functional Movement Specialists (CK-FMSs). You can work with one to correct imbalances and other pre-existing problems that may be reducing your strength and mobility. To find a CK-FMS near you, go to www.dragondoor.com/rkc/ck-fms/.

- For more information about Andrea Du Cane, Master RKC, please visit **www.kettlebellfitness.com**.

References

Vella, C.A. , & Kravitz,L. (2002). Sarcopenia: The mystery of muscle loss. *IDEA Personal Trainer*, 12(4), 30-35.

Balady, GJ., Berra, K.A., Golding, L.A., Gordon, N.F., Mahler, D.A., Myers, J.N., Sheldahl, L.M. (2000). *ACSM's Guidelines for Exercises Testing and Prescription* (Sixth Edition. Lippincott Williams and Wilkins. Evans, W. 1195 Effects of Exercise on Body Composition and Functional Capacity of the Elderly.

M. Bédard, M.M. Porter, S. Marshall, I. Isherwood, J. Riendeau, B. Weaver, H. Tuokko, ... Traffic Injury Prevention 9(1):70-76, 2008. J. Montufar, J. Arango, M.M. Porter, S Nakagawa. ... The effects of strength training on sarcopenia. *Canadian Journal of Applied Physiology*. 26:123-141, 2001

Schoenborn, C. A., Vickerie, J. L., & Powell-Griner, E. (2006). Health characteristics of adults 55 years of age and over: United States, 2000–2003. *Advance Data from Vital and Health Statistics*, (370), 1–32.

Conn, V., Valentine, J., & Cooper, H. (2003). Interventions to increase physical activity among aging adults: A meta-analysis [electronic version]. *Annals of Behavioral Medicine*, 24(3), 190–200.

Get Up and Move: Independence and Maneuverability Related to Regular Exercise among Non-institutionalized Elderly Adults. Author: Heather Soltau Faculty Mentor: James Swan, Department of Applied Gerontology, College of Public Affairs and Community Service Department: Department of Biological Sciences, College of Arts and Sciences & Honors College.

Peterson, M.D. Ph.D., Liberty Athletic Club, Ann Arbor, MI: and Department of Physical Medicine and Rehabilitation, University of Michigan, Ann Arbor, MI, (2010) *Resistance Exercise for Sarcopenic Outcomes and Muscular Fitness in Aging Adults.* NSCA, 32 (3).

About the Author

Andrea Du Cane, Master RKC

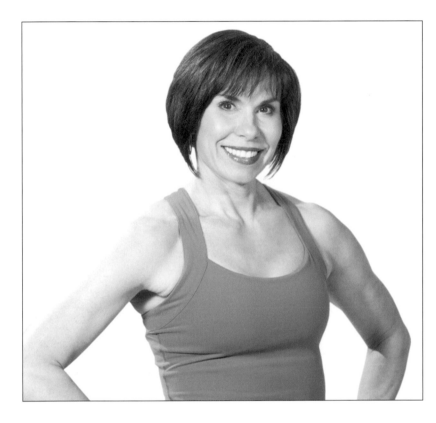

Andrea Du Cane is a Master RKC Instructor and is also CK-FMS certified, CICS and RIST certified, and Z-Health certified. She wrote, produced, and starred in **The Kettlebell Goddess Workout** DVD, and her DVD **Working with Special Populations** was filmed at an RKC Level II workshop. Du Cane was featured in the **From Russia with Tough Love** video and book and the **TRX-Kettlebell** Power DVD. She published an article on Russian kettlebells in *Best Body* Magazine and was interviewed and photographed for an article introducing kettlebells in *Oxygen* magazine.

In addition, Du Cane has a B. A. in Psychology from the University of Minneasota. She is also a Pilates instructor and currently teaches classes in Minneapolis, Minnesota. She has more than 20 years of aerobics, weight training, and fitness experience, with an additional background in several forms of dance, including classical ballet, jazz, and Argentinean tango. She has also trained in a number of Eastern health and martial arts disciplines, including kung fu, yoga, tai chi, and qigong.

"Willful Aging" Declared "Criminally Irresponsible"— Banned in All 50 States...

Reverse Aging, Reduce Pain, Restore Lost Vigor—And Stay Proud of Your Body

Nothing ages us faster than the lack of regular, effective exercise. Muscles melt away, bones go brittle, posture stoops, skin sags, flab hangs—and joints creak. Pain, fear and fatigue become our constant companions.

The less you exercise, the faster you decline. However, not all exercise is created equal. Many forms of exercise may at best put you in a holding pattern, while other forms of exercise might even exacerbate your health issues.

The good news is that there is one form of exercise which can give you immeasurable health benefits, whatever your age. Regular, well-designed **kettlebell workouts** may not only reverse many symptoms of aging, but will actively contribute to building your strength and power well into your 50s, 60s, 70s and 80s.

Discover how the magic of kettlebell exercise can keep you powerful, strong, supple and out of trouble—at any age...

Kettlebells are the only handheld weight that allows you to exercise aerobically, for cardio as well as anaerobically, for strength training. The kettlebell is the unique "gym in your hand" that can reward you with decades of high-yield health benefits.

Andrea Du Cane's *Kettlebell Boomer* presents a complete **De-Aging Masterplan,** that gives everyone from the raw novice to the experienced athlete an opportunity to defy physical decline and hone themselves—safely, simply and progressively—into the muscular, energetic, magnetic specimens they deserve to be.

Kettlebell Boomer provides everything you need to start training with kettlebells—with full instruction plus follow-along workouts. You will discover two main workouts, one with a strength focus and the other cardio. Watch four different people doing the workout, each representing a different level. Pick the right level for you and follow that person through the entire workout. Or you can switch between levels for different exercises.

Bonus sections cover warm-ups, joint mobility, balance and stability—to ensure your anti-aging kettlebell program covers all the essential elements for a long, active, safe and pain-free life. Enjoy!

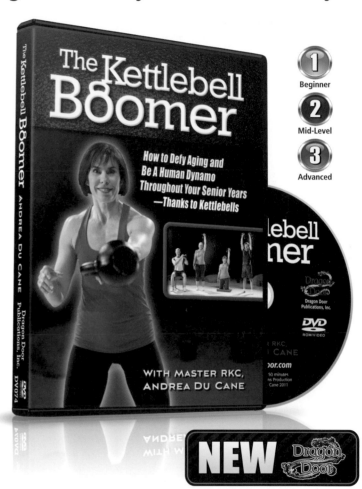

The Kettlebell Boomer
How to Defy Aging and Be a Human Dynamo Throughout Your Senior Years— Thanks to Kettlebells
With Master RKC, Andrea Du Cane
#DV074 $39.95 DVD Running time: 2 hours 50 minutes

DID YOU GET YOUR GODDESS YET?

Reader reviews of Andrea Du Cane's *The Kettlebell Goddess Workout* DVD—Average Rating: 9.11 out of 10 in 123 reviews on dragondoor.com

Finally!!!

"I am so excited about this DVD! I have been training with KB's for three years now off and on, and I have to admit that my motivation has been running low in the past year, and this is just what I needed! Someone to push me, something simple, something sturctured. I have been waiting for a DVD like this for a looong time and now it is finally here! What I like best with it is how it is laid out. It is a complete foolproof way to get your butt kicked a different way each and every day! I love it. And the PDF that came with the DVD shows different ways to schedule your workout or combine different exercises and it gives me absolutely no excuse not to swing that bell! Andrea, great job!" —Ulrika - Detroit, MI

WOW!

"I ordered this DVD before I attended the RKC in September and wow has it given me a new perspective on training. It adds a new excitement on working with KB's. The atmosphere of the DVD creates a relaxing yet motivating theme. I love that

there are different workouts given to help add variety to your training. This DVD is a definite must for men and women, beginners and advanced KBer's."
—Christine Staunch, RKC - Bayonne, NJ

The Complete Package - Astonishing

"If I could I would give this DVD a 20 instead of a 10. Most DVD's only give you a stripped down version of a workout. This marvelous DVD gives you not only 1 workout, like most DVD's. It gives you an infinite amount of them, and they include a warm-up portion and a cool-down routine that is out of this world. These workouts will work you out even if you use a light kettlebell. The instructions are clear cut, and concise for all to understand. Guys will love this DVD as well."—Karen R. Queen - Tampa, Florida

Hard Core Workout!

"Andrea Du Cane provides some tough workouts on The Kettlebell Goddess DVD. This DVD is not for beginners, but it is a great way for someone familiar with basic kettlebell exercises to get a great challenging workout. Each of the goddess workouts are great no-frills, no-nonsense, kick-butt exercise routines. I really enjoy the relax into stretch segment at the end of each workout.

By the way, this DVD is not just for women! My boyfriend loves it as much as I do (though he did complain about not being able to keep up with women wearing pink shirts)."
—Mary - Saratoga, CA

Become the Goddess!!

"WOW!! I purchased this DVD at the RKC in October and I am in LOVE!! I will recommend this DVD to EVERYONE!! This has to be the most kick-butt workout I've tried. My clients will love it! I love the structure of being able to design my own workout with the formulas provided, or just follow along with the workouts already created for us. Andrea - You are awesome! Thanks so much for this DVD! I feel like I'm back at the RKC. (well...almost!)"
—Rae Chitwood, RKC - Mansfield, OH

Excellent!

"This DVD is brilliant! I love the way it is structured to either follow along with the goddess workouts or to create your own. The instruction is great and the workouts are awesome. I can never see myself getting sick of this DVD with all the variety!

I'm newly addicted to kettlebells; I have only be working out with them for a few months now and think this DVD is excellent for beginners. I'd recommend it to both beginners and advanced kettlebellers alike. If you are looking for a serious workout DVD, this is definitely worth it! I love it! I can't thank Andrea enough!!"—Jen - Maine

The Kettlebell Goddess Workout is the Best!

"This is one of the best DVD's that I have ever purchased. It is so complete with workouts and instructions. The variety is terrific. I really enjoyed Andrea in From Russia with Tough Love, but this is best. Nicole and Kristann are a wonderful complement to her and very much inspire me to k working to get better. I tried to just watch the vide without picking up the kettlebells, but I couldn't. I to jump right into a workout. I am glad I did. First t warm up was one of the most thorough that I have ever had. Then the exercises really hit the mark. I h such a pump in my lower body and an overall rush over. Then the nice cool down made me feel like I really accomplished something. I plan to keep on doing the workouts. Thanks for the Kettlebell Godd Workout. Please keep up the good work!" —Robi McGill - Tampa, FL

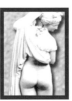

Nothing but positive feedback!!!

"This is a great DVD. I have been getting nothing but positi feedback from my clients. I tried few of them myself and trust n guys, this DVD is not just for the Goddess' but the Gods' can also get worked on the programs as well. The different combinations and ways Andrea shows you how to come up with you own personal routine makes this a must for anyone who wants to get in shape."—Lance Mosley, RKC, CSCS - Palm Beach County, FL

A must have when workin with kettlebells

"This is the best dvd that there is. I received it ab 2 weeks ago and I have been doing it everyday. The really can kick your butt with this dvd. It's a MUST HAVE." —Justine - Downriver MI

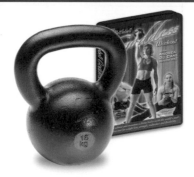

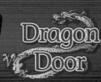

"Stay Strong, Young, Toned and Vibrant With Andrea Du Cane's High-Powered, Super-High-Energy Kettlebell Cardio and Strength Workouts"

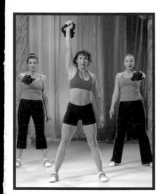

The ancient Greek Goddesses were famous for their vigorous and vibrant strength, their power, their grace and their physical elegance.

Now you have a realistic chance to make even a Greek Goddess green with envy as you match—if not surpass—them for athletic grace and high performance!

In this superbly produced, interactive, menu-based DVD, **Senior Russian Kettlebell Instructor**, *Andrea Du Cane* challenges and inspires you to seize that ideal of elegant strength and make it your own.

Andrea's powerful array of authentic kettlebell workouts, plus cool downs and stretches, are guaranteed to reward you with greater energy, greater well being, greater strength and a superb figure. Fit for the Goddess you know you are!

Choose from a wide variety of **Upper Body, Lower Body, Abs** and **Cardio** workouts, then mix and match to create your own customized training program for godly perfection. Your results will be strictly divine…

Or simply follow along with one of the six **Goddess Workouts** for a complete, carefully targeted session designed to carve away the fat and sculpt lean, toned muscles—ready and willing to take on the world and win it all. Just like Athena… Just like Nike…

Once the hard-kept secret of elite Russian athletes, special forces and 'manly' men, the kettlebell is now becoming the preferred tool for women who are tired of being merely human and tired of mediocre results—and who demand fast fat loss, high energy and exceptional physical performance, now! Let Andrea show you the way…

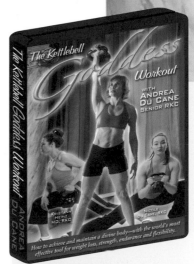

- **Receive** inspiring, first-class personal instruction from one of the nation's top female kettlebell athletes.

  - **Renew** yourself with a constant variety of targeted, high-yield workouts that meet your changing needs.

  - **Redefine** your body and exceed your mortal limits, with the divine challenge of Andrea's patented *Goddess Workouts*.

Includes a **Special Bonus Section** of additional drills to add further variety and power to your workouts.

Contents include a PDF on **How to Get the Most Out of Your** *Kettlebell Goddess Workout* DVD—plus special programming tips.

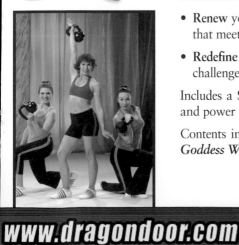

The Kettlebell Goddess Workout

Andrea Du Cane, Master RKC
with Kristann Heinz, MD, RKC and Nicole Du Cane RKC
Running time: 2 Hours and 25 minutes
DVD **#DV040** **$29.95**

1 Beginner
2 Mid-Level

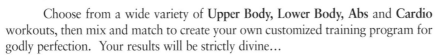

"Kettlebell Training...The Closest Thing You Can Get to Fighting, Without Throwing A Punch"

—Federal Counterterrorist Operator

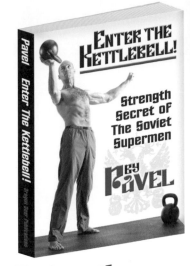

The kettlebell. AK-47 of physical training hardware. Hunk of iron on a handle. Simple, sinister, brutal—and ferociously effective for developing explosive strength, dramatic power and never-say-die conditioning. The man's man's choice for the toughest, most demanding, highest-yield exercise tool on the planet. Guaranteed to forge a rugged, resilient, densely-muscled frame—built to withstand the hardest beating and dish it right back out, 24/7.

Once the prized and jealously-guarded training secret of elite Russian athletes, old-school strongmen and the military, the kettlebell has invaded the West. And taken no prisoners—thanks to former **Soviet Special Forces** physical training instructor and strength author, *Pavel Tsatsouline's* 2001 publication of *The Russian Kettlebell Challenge* and his manufacture of the first traditional Russian kettlebell in modern America.

American hardmen of all stripes were quick to recognize what their Russian counterparts had long known—nothing, nothing beats the kettlebell, when you're looking for a single tool to dramatically impact your strength and conditioning. A storm of success has swept the American S & C landscape, as kettlebell "Comrades" have busted through to new PRs, broken records, thrashed their opponents and elevated their game to new heights of excellence.

With *Enter the Kettlebell!* Pavel delivers a significant upgrade to his original landmark work, *The Russian Kettlebell Challenge*. Drawing on five years of developing and leading the world's first and premiere kettlebell instructor certification program, and after spending five years of additional research into what really works for dramatic results with the kettlebell—we have *Enter the Kettlebell!*

Pavel lays out a foolproof master system that guarantees you success—if you simply follow the commands!

- **Develop** all-purpose strength—to easily handle the toughest and most unexpected demand
- **Maximize** staying power—because the last round decides all
- **Forge** a fighter's physique—because the form must follow the function

Enter the kettlebell! and follow the plan:

1. The New RKC Program Minimum

With just two kettlebell exercises, takes you from raw newbie to solid contender—well-conditioned, flexible, resilient and muscular in all the right places.

2. The RKC Rite of Passage

Jumps you to the next level of physical excellence with Pavel's proven RKC formula for exceptional strength and conditioning.

3. Become a Man Among Men

Propels you to a Special Forces level of conditioning and earns you the right to call yourself a man.

When you rise to the challenge—and *Enter the Kettlebell!*—there will be no more confusion, no more uncertainty and no more excuses—only raw power, never-quit conditioning and earned respect.

Enter the Kettlebell!
Strength Secret of The Soviet Supermen
by Pavel #B33 $34.95
Paperback 200 pages 8.5" x 11"
246 full color photos, charts, and workouts

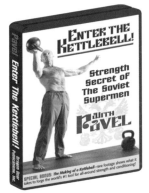

 1 Beginner

 2 Mid-Level

 3 Advanced

DVD with Pavel
#DV036 $29.95
DVD Running time: 46 minutes

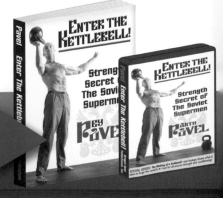

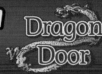

RKC: Premium Kettlebells for a Premium Body!

We Make It Easier for You to Work Hard— With These 3 NEW Military-Grade RKC Kettlebells

By popular demand, we have introduced 3 new RKC kettlebells designed to help women, in particular—but also beginners and smaller men—achieve faster results without greater risk of injury.

Many women told us that the diameter of our traditional **16 kg (35 lb) kettlebell** was unmanageable for their smaller hands. Meaning the grip gave out before they could get the results they otherwise deserved.

The solution? Dragon Door's new, smaller-handled 16 kg RKC kettlebell, which allows our female customers to work out longer and get even greater results.

Again many of our customers— and our instructors—begged us to introduce two new sizes to make it easier to work harder—adding new weight in smaller increments. The solution? Dragon Door's new **10 kg (22 lb)** and **14 kg (31 lb)** RKC kettlebells.

Your Kettlebell Should Last For Ever— And So Should You!

Our 3 new sizes guarantee you decades of solid progress in your strength and conditioning goals.

- **Unique, highly durable paint** prevents ugly rusting and scratching
- **Gorgeous, smooth finish** ensures minimal friction—saves your hands so you can kill your body!
- **Resilient casting job** guarantees a lifetime of hard use in the toughest of terrains
- **Perfect ergonomic design** ensures maximum challenge to the body, while minimizing the chance of injury

Be superior in your preference. Insist that your kettlebell displays the RKC badge of premium quality

10 kg (22 lb)	14 kg (31 lb)	16 kg (35lb)
RKC Kettlebell	**RKC Kettlebell**	**RKC Kettlebell**
#P10T $71.45	**#P10U $87.95**	**#P10S $96.75**

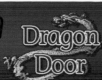

Who trains with kettlebells?

Hard comrades of all persuasions.

Soviet weightlifting legends such as Vlasov, Zhabotinskiy, and Alexeyev started their Olympic careers with old-fashioned kettlebells. Yuri Vlasov once interrupted an interview he was giving to a Western journalist and proceeded to press a pair of kettlebells. "A wonderful exercise," commented the world champion. "...It is hard to find an exercise better suited for developing strength and flexibility simultaneously."

The Russian Special Forces personnel owe much of their wiry strength, explosive agility, and never-quitting stamina to kettlebells. *Soldier, Be Strong!*, the official Soviet armed forces strength training manual pronounced kettlebell drills to be "one of the most effective means of strength development" representing "a new era in the development of human strength-potential".

The elite of the US military and law enforcement instantly recognized the power of the Russian kettlebell, ruggedly simple and deadly effective as an AK-47. You can find Pavel's certified RKC instructors among Force Recon Marines, Department of Energy nuclear security teams, the FBI's Hostage Rescue Team, the Secret Service Counter Assault Team, etc.

Once the Russian kettlebell became a hit among those whose life depends on their strength and conditioning, it took off among hard people from all walks of life: martial artists, athletes, regular hard comrades.

"I can't think of a more practical way of special operations training... I was extremely skeptical about kettlebell training and now wish that I had known about it fifteen years ago..."

—*Name withheld, Special Agent, U.S. Secret Service Counter Assault Team*

Am I kettlebell material?

Kettlebell training is extreme but not elitist. At the 1995 Russian Championship the youngest contestant was 16, the oldest 53! And we are talking elite competition here; the range is even wider if you are training for yourself rather than for the gold. Dr. Krayevskiy, the father of the kettlebell sport, took up training at the age of forty-one and twenty years later he was said to look fresher and healthier than at forty.

Only 8.8% of top Russian gireviks, members of the Russian National Team and regional teams, reported injuries in training or competition (Voropayev, 1997). A remarkably low number, especially if you consider that these are elite athletes who push their bodies over the edge. Many hard men with high mileage have overcome debilitating injuries with kettlebell training (get your doctor's approval). Acrobat Valentin Dikul fell and broke his back at seventeen. Today, in his mid-sixties, he juggles 180-pound balls and breaks powerlifting records!

"... kettlebells are a unique conditioning tool and a powerful one as well that you should add to your arsenal of strength... my experience with them has been part of what's led me to a modification in my thoughts on strength and bodyweight exercises... I'm having a blast training with them and I think you will as well."

—Bud Jeffries, the author of *How to Squat 900lbs. without Drugs, Powersuits, or Kneewraps*

How do I learn to use the kettlebell?

From Pavel's books and videos: *The Russian Kettlebell Challenge* or *From Russia with Tough Love* for comrades ladies. From an RKC certified instructor; find one in your area on RussianKettlebell.com. Kettlebell technique can be learned in one or two sessions and you can start intense training during the second or even first week (Dvorkin, 2001).

"...I felt rejuvenated and ready to conquer the world. I was sold on the kettlebells, as the exercises were fun and challenging, and demanded coordination, explosion, balance, and power... I am now on my way to being a better, fitter, and more explosive grappler, and doing things I haven't done in years!"

—Kid Peligro, *Grappling* magazine

What is the right kettlebell size for me?

Kettlebells come in 'poods'. A pood is an old Russian measure of weight, which equals 16kg, or roughly 35 lbs. An average man should start with a 35-pounder. It does not sound like a lot but believe it; it feels a lot heavier than it should! Most men will eventually progress to a 53-pounder, the standard issue size in the Russian military. Although available in most units, 70-pounders are used only by a few advanced guys and in elite competitions. 88-pounders are for mutants.

An average woman should start with an 18-pounder. A strong woman can go for a 26-pounder. Some women will advance to a 35-pounder. A few hard women will go beyond.

"Kettlebells are like weightlifting times ten."

"Kettlebells are like weightlifting times ten. ...If I could've met Pavel in the early '80s, I might've won two gold medals. I'm serious."

—Dennis Koslowski, D.C., RKC, *Olympic Silver Medalist in Greco-Roman Wrestling*

Classic RKC Kettlebells (Cast Iron/E-Coated)

Item	Weight	Price	MAIN USA	PUERTO RICO	AK&HI	CAN
#P10N	10 lb	$37.95	S/H $14.00	$47.00	$53.00	$35.00
#P10P	14 lb	$49.95	S/H $16.00	$51.00	$57.00	$41.00
#P10M	18 lb	$59.95	S/H $22.00	$65.00	$71.00	$46.00
#P10T	10 kg (22 lb)	$64.95	S/H $25.00	$73.00	$79.00	$52.00
#P10G	12 kg (27 lb)	$69.95	S/H $28.00	$80.00	$86.00	$58.00
#P10U	14 kg (31 lb)	$79.95	S/H $34.00	$93.00	$99.00	$64.00
#P10A	16 kg (36 lb)	$87.95	S/H $38.00	$104.00	$110.00	$72.00
#P10S (Women's)	16 kg (36 lb)	$87.95	S/H $38.00	$104.00	$110.00	$72.00
#P10H	20 kg (45 lb)	$97.95	S/H $44.00	$123.00	$122.00	$85.00
#P10B	24 kg (53 lb)	$107.95	S/H $49.00	$141.00	$139.00	$94.00
#P10J	28 kg (62 lb)	$129.95	S/H $53.00	$162.00	$157.00	$107.00
#P10C	32 kg (71 lb)	$139.95	S/H $55.00	$186.00	$193.00	$121.00
#P10Q	36 kg (80 lb)	$159.95	S/H $58.00	$203.00	$209.00	$134.00
#P10F	40 kg (89 lb)	$179.95	S/H $64.00	$223.00	$229.00	$148.00
#P10R	44 kg (97 lb)	$219.95	S/H $69.00	$241.00	$247.00	$160.00
#P10L	48 kg (106 lb)	$239.95	S/H $75.00	$261.00	$267.00	$175.00

SAVE! ORDER A SET OF CLASSIC KETTLEBELLS & SAVE $$$

	Item	Weight	Price	MAIN USA	PUERTO RICO	AK&HI	CAN
Save $15.00	#SP10	Classic Set—35, 53 & 70 lb.	$320.85	S/H $142.00	$431.00	$450.00	$287.00
Save $15.00	#SP11	Women's Set—10, 14 & 18 lb.	$132.85	S/H $52.00	$163.00	$181.00	$122.00

ALASKA/HAWAII KETTLEBELL ORDERING
Dragon Door now ships to all 50 states, including Alaska and Hawaii, via UPS Ground.

CANADIAN KETTLEBELL ORDERING
Dragon Door now accepts online, phone and mail orders for Kettlebells to Canada, using UPS Standard service. UPS Standard to Canada service is guaranteed, fully tracked ground delivery, available to every address in all of Canada's ten provinces. Delivery time can vary between 3 to 10 days.

IMPORTANT – International shipping quotes & orders do not include customs clearance, duties, taxes or other non-routine customs brokerage charges, which are the responsibility of the customer.

- KETTLEBELLS ARE SHIPPED VIA UPS GROUND SERVICE, UNLESS OTHERWISE REQUESTED.
- KETTLEBELLS RANGING IN SIZE FROM 4KG TO 24KG CAN BE SHIPPED TO P.O. BOXES OR MILITARY ADDDRESSES VIA THE U.S. POSTAL SERVICE, BUT WE REQUIRE PHYSICAL ADDDRESSES FOR UPS DELIVERIES FOR THE 32KG AND 40KG KETTLEBELLS.
- **NO** RUSH ORDERS ON KETTLEBELLS!

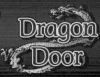

www.dragondoor.com
1·800·899·5111

Dragon Door

Order Dragon Door Kettlebells online:
dragondoor.com/shop-by-department/kettlebells/

Men, New to Kettlebells? Here's How to Get the Fastest and Most Effective Strength, Conditioning and Fat-Loss Results with Your Russian Kettlebell...

The kettlebell is the world's single most effective tool for rapid fat loss, fast strength gains and unbeatable endurance. However, in order to properly and fully reap these benefits from your kettlebell, we strongly recommend you properly educate yourself in how to use the kettlebell correctly.

Pavel Tsatsouline is the fitness expert and author who has single-handedly introduced the United States to the powerful physical benefits of kettlebells. So the best way to ensure you get optimal results is to absorb Pavel's advice from his groundbreaking book and companion DVD, *Enter the Kettlebell!*

Pavel's *Enter the Kettlebell!* book gives you the theory, detailed instructions and superb photography to ensure you know exactly what you are doing. Pavel's *Enter the Kettlebell!* DVD supplies that crucial ingredient that you simply can't expect to get from a book alone— the three-dimensional movement that fully illustrates the correct trajectories and other key elements that only film can communicate.

So, we have put together quick-start kits that incorporate all three of these resources, with your choice of three different weight sizes. (And you save $10.00 over the investment if you paid for these items individually.)

Special Men's Kettlebell Quick-Start Kits Help Save You Money, Shed Pounds... Gain Muscle, Power And Energy!

The best weight for a man of average strength to begin with is our

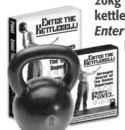

16kg or 35-pound kettlebell with Pavel's *Enter the Kettlebell!* **book and DVD**

Men's 35lb Russian Kettlebell Quick-Start Kit

Item **#KKB009** **$145.49** plus $43.50 SH

The best weight for a strong man to begin with is our

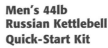

20kg or 44-pound kettlebell with Pavel's *Enter the Kettlebell!* **book and DVD**

Men's 44lb Russian Kettlebell Quick-Start Kit

Item **#KKB014** **$155.39** plus $50.50 SH

The best weight for a very strong man to begin with is our

24kg or 53-pound kettlebell with Pavel's *Enter the Kettlebell!* **book and DVD**

Men's 53lb Russian Kettlebell Quick-Start Kit

Item **#KKB015** **$165.47** plus $54.50 SH

Save On Your Total Kettlebell Investment When You Purchase a Pair of Same-Weight Kettlebells

X2

CLASSIC KETTLEBELL PAIRS (SOLID CAST IRON/E-COATING)

ORDER A PAIR & SAVE $10.00		Price	MAIN USA	PUERTO RICO	AK&HI	CAN
#P10TA	Two 10 kg (22 lb)	$128.60	S/H $50.00	$146.00	$158.00	$104.00
#P10GA	Two 12 kg (27 lb)	$138.50	S/H $56.00	$160.00	$172.00	$116.00
#P10UA	Two 14 kg (31 lb)	$158.30	S/H $68.00	$168.00	$198.00	$128.00
#P10AA	Two 16 kg (36 lb)	$174.15	S/H $76.00	$208.00	$220.00	$144.00
#P10HA	Two 20 kg (45 lb)	$193.94	S/H $88.00	$246.00	$260.00	$170.00
#P10BA	Two 24 kg (53 lb)	$213.74	S/H $98.00	$282.00	$294.00	$188.00
#P10JA	Two 28 kg (62 lb)	$257.30	S/H $106.00	$324.00	$336.00	$214.00
#P10CA	Two 32 kg (71 lb)	$277.10	S/H $110.00	$372.00	$386.00	$242.00

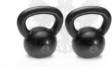
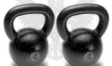
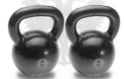
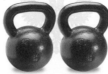
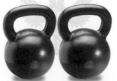
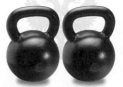

www.dragondoor.com
1-800-899-5111

Dragon Door

Order Dragon Door Kettlebells online: dragondoor.com/shop-by-department/kettlebells/

Be Flexible Like a Young Child—yet Move with Strength and Speed

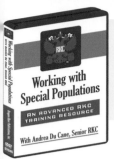

How to REGAIN Your Range-of-Motion, RESTORE Mobility and RENEW Your Energy...

Working with Special Populations

An Advanced RKC Training Resource
With Andrea Du Cane, Master RKC

Running Time: 2 hours 57 minutes

2-DVD set   #DV046   *$77.00*

Are you "broken", suffering from high mileage or fighting unsuccessfully with some stubborn physical challenge? Or do you have clients who are struggling with serious dysfunction?

As a Master RKC Andrea Du Cane has helped hundreds of her clients break through their particular physical challenges—and live more vigorous, accomplished lives.

Discover a multitude of methods to address corrective, preventive and restorative issues for your clients—or for yourself.

Are You Quitting—Because You Hurt Too Much?

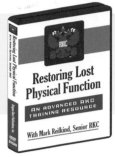

How to End the Pain and Spring Back into Action

Restoring Lost Physical Function

An Advanced RKC Training Resource
With Mark Reifkind, Senior RKC

Running Time: 117 minutes

2-DVD set   #DV048   *$77.00*

A series of brutal injuries ended Mark Reifkind's Olympic hopes in gymnastics, in champion powerlifting, in ultra-marathons and in Ironman triathlons. A resurgent Mark battled back to become one of the premier kettlebell trainers in the US.

No one has delved more deeply than Mark into what it takes to beat pain at its own game—and remain resiliently functional in the face of the most egregious challenges.

In a brilliant, inspiring, impassioned, fascinating and highly practical seminar, Mark blows us away with his methods for understanding, pinpointing and then releasing blocks in the body.

Dramatically Improve Athletic Performance and Safely Extend Your Career

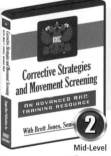

How PROFESSIONALS identify and FIX imbalances in their body to avoid injury...

Corrective Strategies & Movement Screening

An Advanced RKC Training Resource
By Brett Jones, Master RKC

Running Time: 3 hours 2 minutes

2-DVD set   #DV047   *$77.00*

▶▶ What is a Corrective Strategy?
▶▶ Movement Screening — The Functional Movement Screen for Kettlebells
▶▶ Basic history — injury, medical, exercise, sports/activity
▶▶ Clearance screens — Neck, Shoulder and Back
▶▶ Basic screens —Toe Touch, Single leg stance, Active Straight Leg Raise
▶▶ Movement Screens — Deep squat, In-line Lunge, Shoulder Mobility and
  ▶▶ Trunk Stability Push-up
  ▶▶ Shoulder/Thoracic spine corrections, Stability work and Deep squat progression

---

End the indignity and shame of modern-day softness

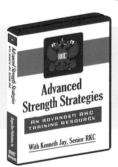

The ultimate protocol for building a JACK-HAMMER HEART and the INVINCIBLE HARDINESS of an ancient warrior

Advanced Strength Strategies

An Advanced RKC Training Resource
With Kenneth Jay, Senior RKC

Running Time: One hour 42 minutes

2-DVD set   #DV049   *$77.00*

With pointers, charts, diagrams, stats and wads of research to back him up, Kenneth Jay delivers convincing proof that a carefully calculated, personalized kettlebell snatch protocol can give us the most outstanding cardio of our lives. And give us a fighting chance to be mentioned in the same breath as those immensely powerful warriors of ancient times.

The Level II RKCs got a thorough schooling in Cardiovascular Kettlebell Concepts and how to massively enhance their all-important VO2Max.

RKC Level II Advanced Training Series

Look WAY YOUNGER than Your Age, Have a LEAN, GRACEFUL, Athletic-Looking Body, Feel AMAZING, Feel VIGOROUS, Feel BEAUTIFUL, Have MORE Energy and MORE Strength to, Get MORE Done in Your Day

In Russia, kettlebells have long been revered as the fitness-tool of choice for Olympic athletes, elite special forces and martial artists. The kettlebell's ballistic movement challenges the body to achieve an unparalleled level of physical conditioning and overall strength.

But until now, the astonishing benefits of the Russian kettlebell have been unavailable to all but a few women. Kettlebells have mostly been the sacred preserve of the male professional athlete, the military and other hardcore types. That's about to change, as Russian fitness expert and best selling author PAVEL, delivers the first-ever kettlebell program for women.

It's wild, but women really CAN have it all when they access the magical power of Russian kettlebells. Pavel's uncompromising workouts give *across-the-board, simultaneous, spectacular and immediate results* for all aspects of physical fitness: strength, speed, endurance, fat-burning, you name it. Kettlebells deliver any and everything a woman could want—if she wants to be in the best-shape-ever of her life.

And one handy, super-simple tool—finally available in woman-friendly sizes—does it all. No bulky, expensive machines. No complicated gizmos. No time-devouring trips to the gym.

Into sports? Jump higher. Leap further. Kick faster. Hit harder. Throw harder. Run with newfound speed. Swim with greater power. Endure longer. Wow!

Working hard? Handle stress with ridiculous ease. Blaze thru tasks in half the time. Radiate confidence. Knock 'em dead with your energy and enthusiasm.

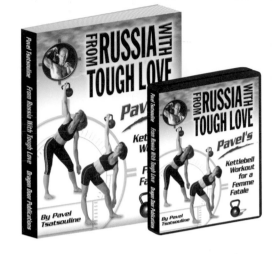

From Russia with Tough Love

Pavel's Kettlebell Workout for a Femme Fatale
With Pavel Tsatsouline
Running Time: 1hr 12 minutes
DVD #DV002 $29.95

1 Beginner

2 Mid-Level

By Pavel Tsatsouline
Paperback   184 pages   8.5" x 11"
Book   #B22 $34.95

From Russia with Tough Love Book and DVD Set

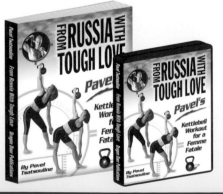

Item #DVS005 $59.90

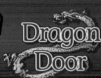

Purchase Pavel's From Russia With Tough Love book and DVD as a set and save...

How to stay informed of the latest advances in strength and conditioning
Visit http://kbforum.dragondoor.com/

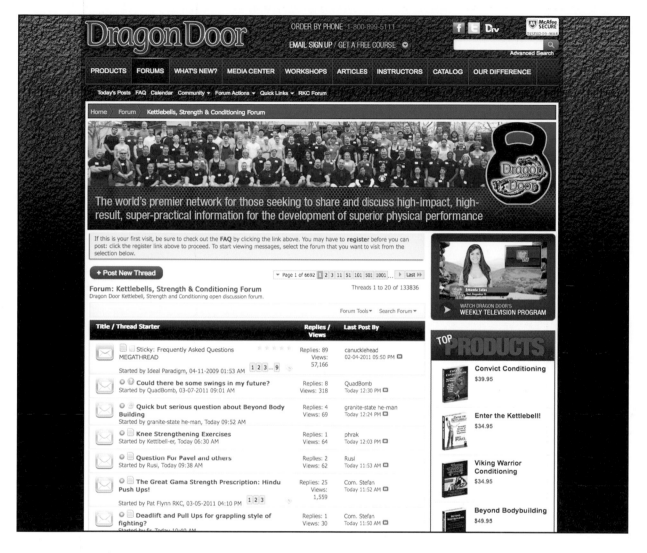

Visit www.dragondoor.com for late-breaking news and tips on how to stay ahead of the fitness pack.

Visit http://kbforum.dragondoor.com/ and participate in Dragon Door's stimulating and informative **Strength and Conditioning** Forum. Post your fitness questions or comments and get quick feedback from Pavel Tsatsouline and other leading fitness experts.

Visit www.dragondoor.com and browse the **Articles** section and other pages for groundbreaking theories and products for improving your health and well being.

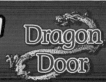

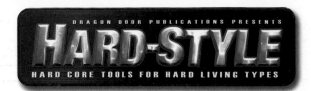

1·800·899·5111
24 HOURS A DAY
FAX YOUR ORDER (866) 280-7619

ORDERING INFORMATION

Customer Service Questions? Please call us between 9:00am– 11:00pm EST Monday to Friday at 1-800-899-5111. Local and foreign customers call 513-346-4160 for orders and customer service

100% One-Year Risk-Free Guarantee. If you are not completely satisfied with any product—we'll be happy to give you a prompt exchange, credit, or refund, as you wish. Simply return your purchase to us,

and please let us know why you were dissatisfied—it will help us to provide better products and services in the future. *Shipping and handling fees are non-refundable.*

Telephone Orders For faster service you may place your orders by calling Toll Free 24 hours a day, 7 days a week, 365 days per year. When you call, please have your credit card ready.

Complete and mail with full payment to: Dragon Door Publications, 5 County Road B East, Suite 3, Little Canada, MN 55117

Please print clearly

Sold To: A

Name_____

Street_____

City_____

State _____ Zip _____

Day phone*_____
* Important for clarifying questions on orders

Please print clearly

SHIP TO: *(Street address for delivery)*   B

Name_____

Street_____

City_____

State _____ Zip _____

Email_____

Warning to foreign customers:
The Customs in your country may or may not tax or otherwise charge you an additional fee for goods you receive. Dragon Door Publications is charging you only for U.S. handling and international shipping. Dragon Door Publications is in no way responsible for any additional fees levied by Customs, the carrier or any other entity.

ITEM #	QTY.	ITEM DESCRIPTION	ITEM PRICE	A OR B	TOTAL

HANDLING AND SHIPPING CHARGES • NO COD'S
Total Amount of Order Add (Excludes kettlebells and kettlebell kits):

$00.00 to 29.99	Add $6.00	$100.00 to 129.99	Add $14.00
$30.00 to 49.99	Add $7.00	$130.00 to 169.99	Add $16.00
$50.00 to 69.99	Add $8.00	$170.00 to 199.99	Add $18.00
$70.00 to 99.99	Add $11.00	$200.00 to 299.99	Add $20.00
		$300.00 and up	Add $24.00

Canada and Mexico add $6.00 to US charges. All other countries, flat rate, double US Charges. See Kettlebell section for Kettlebell Shipping and handling charges.

Total of Goods	
Shipping Charges	
Rush Charges	
Kettlebell Shipping Charges	
OH residents add 6.5% sales tax	
MN residents add 6.5% sales tax	
TOTAL ENCLOSED	

METHOD OF PAYMENT ❑ CHECK ❑ M.O. ❑ MASTERCARD ❑ VISA ❑ DISCOVER ❑ AMEX

Account No. *(Please indicate all the numbers on your credit card)*   EXPIRATION DATE

☐☐☐☐ ☐☐☐☐ ☐☐☐☐ ☐☐☐☐   ☐☐/☐☐

Day Phone: (   )_____

Signature: _____   **Date:** _____

NOTE: *We ship best method available for your delivery address. Foreign orders are sent by air. Credit card or International M.O. only. For* **RUSH** *processing of your order, add an additional $10.00 per address. Available on money order & charge card orders only.*

Errors and omissions excepted. Prices subject to change without notice.